# *101* Ways
## to Use
# Noni Fruit Juice
## For Your Better Health

A Handbook of Oral, Topical and

Internal Applications and Procedures

## Isa Navarre

Direct Source Publishing
15 East 400 South
Orem, Utah 84058
U.S.A.

**101 Ways to Use Noni Fruit Juice for Your Better Health**
**A Handbook of Oral, Topical and Internal Applications and Procedures**
Copyright © 2005 Isa Navarre

Cover Design by Shane Allman Art & Design.
Back Cover Photo by Robert Morton.

Printed in the United States of America.
ISBN 13: 978-1-933057-24-8
ISBN 10: 1-933057-24-6

**– IMPORTANT NOTICE –**
The information in this book is designed to provide health information for purposes of reference and guidance and to accompany, not replace, the services of a qualified health care practitioner or physician. It is not the intent of the author or publisher to prescribe any substance to cure, mitigate, treat, or prevent any disease. In the event you use this information with or without seeking medical attention, the author and publisher shall not be liable or otherwise responsible for any loss, damage or injury caused by or arising out of, directly or indirectly, the information contained in this book or its use.

# -DEDICATION-

My daughter, Aria Ray, was born two weeks after I started taking Noni fruit juice. The idea for this book came soon afterwards. I felt it was significant that her birth, my introduction to Noni, and the idea for this book happened so closely together. In ancient Polynesia, knowledge of healing was conveyed from one generation to the next. This book will help me follow that tradition, as well as introduce Noni to families all over the world. I feel very blessed to be part of that. And so, I dedicate this book to children everywhere, and in particular, to Aria Ray and Kellan, my daughters who were born since I began taking Noni.

# -TABLE OF CONTENTS-

**SECTION 2**

# -ACKNOWLEDGEMENTS-

To all of my readers, I offer a deep and heartfelt "thank you." This book would not be possible without you. Your love for Noni and interest in knowing more about how to work with it has kept me collecting ways to use Noni since 1996. It is always my honor and privilege to share with you what I have discovered.

Today one of my daughters learned that when a gift is received a gift is returned. Life ensures the equation is perfect and perpetuated. She saw the principle in action when she returned a kind act with a smile of love that became a gift to the giver of the kind act, who then felt all the more love for her. So she entered a circle of gratitude.

Nature gives us the gift of Noni. We receive it with open hearts and our gratitude goes out into life. Life returns the gift back to us and our bodies respond with greater harmony and well-being. Our bodies, then, also deserve acknowledgement. Their health challenges can lead us into a circle of gratitude that includes everyone in the world who is also thankful for Noni. We are uplifted by a common experience and the gratitude felt by all.

Special thanks to the pickers, producers and distributors of Noni fruit juice; and to the publisher of this book; to Paul and McKinley, who invited me to write it; and to Connie, for her friendship and for providing me with Noni.

# -FOREWORD-

During the first half of the 20ᵗʰ Century, a great deal of common-sense health care information was lost as our country went through the institutionalization and industrialization of medicine. This resulted in large segments of the population putting their care (along with their personal choices and power), into the hands of physicians, pharmaceutical companies, and technology.

The second half of this century, it seems, has been a reclaiming of our common-sense knowledge, personal choices, and personal power. This process of reclamation has come in waves, each wave growing as new waves developed.

The first wave was a growing awareness of the importance of good foods, then came the wave of vitamins and minerals, then the wave of phytonutrients (antioxidants, alkaloids, glucopolysaccharides, etc.), and herbs. I believe that Noni fruit juice exemplifies the crest of this latest wave. Phytonutrients represent a step beyond what we traditionally call "vitamins." They are specialized plant compounds that have beneficial functions in our bodies. Examples of good sources of phytonutrients you may already be familiar with include ginseng, licorice, ginkgo biloba, and aloe vera.

Noni fruit juice is known to contain many different kinds of phytonutrients. These include a glucopolysaccharide that is known to boost the immune system, a compound that can inhibit viruses and cancerous changes in DNA, and the precursor to an alkaloid called xeronine that improves the functioning of your enzymes and cell wall receptors. These compounds work together to boost each other's effectiveness.

And, they have been designed and formulated by the wisdom of nature rather than by someone in a laboratory. I have been working in the field of conventional, nutritional, and alternative medicine for twelve years and I have not seen another natural substance as interesting and widely effective as Noni fruit juice.

Optimal functioning of your immune system is vital to your overall wellness, every biochemical reaction in your body utilizes enzymes and all of your cellular communication mechanisms use cell wall receptors. Because Noni fruit juice works on such basic levels, you can well imagine that it has many uses. And, indeed, this is what we see clinically. I have used Noni fruit juice in my practice since October, 1996, and have seen dramatic results in hundreds of people. I have talked with yet hundreds more from all around the Country who are also seeing dramatic results from Noni fruit juice.

The concept of Noni fruit juice is simple. It is just a juice. And it is as safe for you as orange juice or apple juice. So how could it have so many powerful therapeutic benefits? After all, in our pharmacological culture, don't powerful therapies belong in the domain of physicians and aren't they known to have powerful side-effects? Can't people hurt themselves with a powerful therapy if they don't know what they are doing?

Generally, yes, but think about it this way. If you were severely deficient in vitamin C, you would have a condition called scurvy. Vitamin C, among other things, helps with the production of collagen, the main ingredient in our connective tissue. So scurvy is a condition where your body is literally falling apart. If you had scurvy, a glass of orange juice would have powerful therapeutic benefits. A glass or two of orange juice per day would prevent it altogether, and you would have to drink a tremendous amount of orange juice to hurt yourself.

The analogy applies to Noni in that many of us are severely xeronine deficient. Nutrient-depleted soils, environmental pollution, the stress of everyday life, aging, diseases, and certain food additives all work together to deplete our xeronine.

Noni fruit juice supplies the necessary nutrients so that our bodies can make more xeronine.

As with other nutrients, herbs, or remedies, the more you know about Noni fruit juice, the more you can obtain its full benefits. This is the power and beauty of this book—that it can help you understand the wide range of applications of Noni fruit juice. When I first read *53 Ways to Use Noni Fruit Juice*, [now *101 Ways to Use Noni*], even after a year of using Noni fruit juice myself and in my practice, many of the concepts and applications were new to me. And I have to admit, I was somewhat skeptical. But I tried some of the suggestions myself and recommended others to patients and watched what happened. Now I am a believer.

I think that Isa Navarre has successfully synthesized intuitive and experimental science to bring us this straightforward yet comprehensive guide to the many uses of Noni fruit juice. I expect that this book will help you receive even more benefit from this juice, this amazing gift from God.

Steven M. Hall, M.D.
January 5, 1998

# -What You Should Know About Noni Juice-

Since 1996, when Noni fruit juice first became commercially available, many Noni products have found their way to the marketplace. Most are powdered and in capsules and others are liquid. Of the liquid ones, some are the pure extract of the Noni fruit, and others are reconstituted from dried or powdered fruit. A few also contain extracts of the roots and leaves of the Noni plant.

In researching this book, I used juice that is a pure extract of the Noni fruit. It contains the natural, perfect mix of the pulpy and the watery part of the fruit. This is important because these two fruit components have unique properties. Together, they are a dynamic pair.

I also feel it is important to know where the Noni that you use comes from. Noni grows in practically all tropical regions of the world, from Puerto Rico to India. However, the soils of the world are not the same. The best Noni grows in unspoiled, nutrient-rich, volcanic soil—such as that of the remote Polynesian islands in the South Pacific. Juice from this Noni fruit has unsurpassed purity and an abundance of beneficial compounds. Both these factors are critical to fully benefit from the applications in this book.

Please feel welcome to experiment with Noni fruit juice. Try a few of the procedures in this book. Customize them to suit your individual needs. Get to know Noni by finding out how your body responds to different dosages. Which topical applications help you the most? Noni can become a life-long family friend.

Read on, and allow me to introduce you...

# -INTRODUCTION-

## HOW MY EXPERIENCES
## WITH NONI BEGAN:

"My cells remember this," I exclaimed moments after drinking my first ounce of Noni fruit juice. Somehow, Noni felt familiar. A few minutes later, changes started happening in my body. I was in my last month of pregnancy and the heartburn I had been suffering subsided. I felt more calm and peaceful, and a tight muscle in my back suddenly released. I continued to take two ounces of Noni daily and the premature labor contractions I was having never came back. I was able to get out of bed and enjoy my last month of pregnancy walking around, working, and enjoying life.

Obviously, Noni was special. Of all the nutritional supplements I had tried over the years, nothing was as versatile and effective as Noni. I began to experiment with myself and my family, and was amazed at all the ways that Noni proved helpful.

Although it is better to take Noni on an empty stomach, the Noni Antacid Substitute, which is taken after a meal, did wonders for my indigestion. I also used Noni Massage Oil to help prevent stretch-marks and prepared Noni Tea to boost my immune system for the upcoming labor.

On October 30th, 1996, I gave birth to an eight-pound baby girl, named Aria Ray. My afterbirth cramps were very painful. Frequent Noni Compresses helped not only to reduce the pain, but also to heal the stitches I had received. A Trauma Serving sped my recovery, and a Maintenance Serving of two ounces a day helped me produce abundant milk to feed my baby. Later, Noni Nose Drops cleared her stuffy nose. The Noni Tummy

Treatment helped her body overcome a fever, and the Noni Rash Plaster quickly took care of an occasional diaper rash.

Noni Ear Drops have helped all my children beat ear infections. The Noni Mini-Compress and First Aid for Minor Wounds has helped everyone in my family. We have been amazed at how quickly Noni has sped our recovery from cuts, scrapes, burns and scratches.

## MY FAMILY'S MIRACLE:

In the summer of 1996, our German Shepherd dog, Aka, became severely ill. His hair fell out, and he scratched and chewed his body until it bled. Conventional treatment made him worse, and herbal and homeopathic remedies helped only a little.

In November, I tried giving him Noni. I followed the Procedure for Serious Conditions and every two weeks Interrupted his Noni Regimen for a day or two. Twice a day I applied the Noni Topical Splash to his lesions. Five times a day, I used a plastic syringe to inject an ounce of Noni into his mouth. He was very good about it. Maybe he knew it would help him feel better.

It did. By January he was completely healed. All his hair had grown back—in fact, it looked shinier and healthier than before. He also regained his playful joy for living. Our whole family was so grateful for Noni!

## WHY NONI WORKS:

Although this book focuses on the myriad ways to use Noni, I wanted to touch on why Noni works. Researchers have identified over one-hundred-fifty compounds in the *Morinda citrifolia*, or Noni fruit, which have therapeutic value.[1]  Two of

---

[1]  Neil Solomon, M.D. Ph.D., *Noni Juice: How Much How Often for What* (Vineyard: Direct Source Publishing, 2004), pp. 2, 3.

these compounds (anthraquinones and scopoletin), have been proven to be helpful against bacteria, fungus, inflammation, and allergies.[2] Another compound (terpenes), which is also found in essential oils, helps rejuvenate cells.[3] French scientists had success testing Noni's painkilling elements.[4] Japanese researchers found a compound (damnacanthal) that inhibited pre-cancerous cells.[5] And Dr. Ralph Heinicke, who received his Ph.D. in biochemistry from the University of Minnesota, discovered that Noni contains an appreciable quantity of a compound that he identified and named "proxeronine."[6]

Proxeronine helps the body make an important alkaloid that Dr. Heinicke also discovered, which he called "xeronine." Xeronine is very important to the body because it regulates and strengthens the protein in our cells. Protein is found everywhere in our body and does many things. For example, proteins comprise the bulk of the organic material within the cell. Hemoglobin, insulin, collagen, as well as muscle and skin, cell membranes, blood vessel walls, blood clots, enzymes and many hormones are also made of protein.[7] Xeronine's impact on protein may help to explain Noni's effectiveness for so many different conditions.[8]

Studies on the various compounds found in the Noni plant continue to this day and more research papers are published every year.

If you would like to read more about Noni's ingredients and studies which have been done on Noni, may I suggest the books, *Noni Juice: How Much How Often for What,* by Neil Solomon, M.D. Ph.D., *Noni—Polynesia's Natural Pharmacy,* and *Noni (Morinda citrifolia) Prize Herb of the South Pacific.* These books are available from Direct Source by calling toll free 1-800-748-2996.

[2]  *Noni—Polynesia's Natural Pharmacy* (Vineyard: Pride Publishing, 1997), pp. 17, 18.

[3]  Julia Morton, "The Ocean-Going Noni, or Indian Mulberry and Some of Its Colorful Relatives," *Economic Botany,* Vol. 46 (3), 1992.

[4]  Chafique Younos, Alain Rolland, Jacques Fleurentin, Marie-Claire Lanhers, Rene Misslin, and Francois Mortier, "Analgesic and Behavioral Effects of *Morinda citrifolia,"* *Planta Med.,* Vol. 56, 1990.

[5]  Tomonori Hiramatsu, Masaya Imoto, Takashi Koyano, Kazuo Umezawa, "Induction of Normal Phenotypes in *Ras*-Transformed Cells by Damnacanthal from *Morinda citrifolia,"* *Cancer Letters,* Vol. 75, 1993.

[6]  R.M. Heinicke, "The Pharmacologically Active Ingredient of Noni," *Pacific Tropical Botanical Garden Bulletin,* Vol. 15, No. 1, January 1985.

[7]  Fleur L. Strand, *Physiology: A Regulatory Systems Approach,* (New York: Macmillan, 1978), pp. 31, 56, 57, 65.

[8]  R.M. Heinicke, "The Pharmacologically Active Ingredient of Noni," *Pacific Tropical Botanical Garden Bulletin,* Vol. 15, No. 1, January 1985.

# FROM 53 WAYS TO 78 WAYS TO 101 WAYS:

Soon after I was introduced to Noni fruit juice, I began to record the many ways I was using Noni. This resulted in the book, *53 Ways to Use Noni*. Since then, I heard from Noni enthusiasts around the world about how these techniques helped them. They also offered new ideas for using Noni, which I added to my growing repertoire. In November, 2000, I felt that I had gathered enough new "ways" that I could expand the book. This was how the previous edition, *78 Ways to Use Noni*, evolved.

Then in the spring of 2005, the publisher contacted me about the possibility of updating *78 Ways*. I thought the least I could do was reedit it. But when I sat down to list other ways to use Noni based on my experiences over the past few years, I came up with about twenty within a few minutes. In the process of rewriting the book, several more emerged until I ended up with 101.

Since *78 Ways* was published, by far the most frequent question I've been asked is how to use Noni more economically. New chapters that address this question include The Maintenance Economy Serving, Enhancing Noni's Effects with Water and The Sipping Method for Finding Your Ideal Amount. Appendix A now lists all the ways in this book that enhance Noni's effects and many of them can be used in combination.

Essential to the question of economy is knowing how well Noni is working for you. If you are having great results, the price is worth every penny. Three chapters now address how to evaluate Noni. The Noni Health Evaluation Sheets, once a part of the appendix, are updated and are now included in the book along with chapters on Evaluating Your Progress with Noni and How to Achieve Your Health Goals with Noni. These chapters contain ways to chart your progress towards greater health with Noni.

Other new methods for boosting Noni's effects include The Busy Person's Way to Enhance their Daily Serving, and Using Intention with Noni. New methods for incorporating Noni into daily living include the Family Serving, the Sick-Day Prevention Serving, and Noni as a Sleep Aid.  A few of the new topical applications include the Noni Abdominal Conditioner, A Noni Procedure for ailing joints, Easy Noni Skin Conditioner, Noni for the Immune System and more.

Again, this is just a sample of the new ways to use Noni that you will find in this book. I also took the liberty to rename some procedures to better reflect their purpose.  The Maintenance Serving #2 is now "Getting Comfortable with Noni;" Maintenance Serving #3 was renamed "The Anti-Stress Procedure;" Maintenance Serving #4 evolved into two chapters, "The Maintenance Economy Serving" and "Enhancing Noni's Effects with Water;" the Small Area Treatment is now "The Noni Mini-Compress;" and the Noni Fast Method #3 is now the "Noni Detoxification Program."

You will also find new versions of the Noni Facial, the Noni Back Compress, Noni Eye Drops and the Trauma Serving.

Those who are familiar with *78 Ways* will find many changes in this book.  There are updates, revisions, clarifications, expansions and new versions of several techniques.  Even the few chapters that are basically unchanged received editing for clarity.  I've also put the chapters in Section 1 into what seems a more logical order.

The Table of Contents will give you the best overview of what you can find in this book, and the index will guide you to specific information you may be looking for.

## HOW TO USE THIS BOOK:

I have divided the 101 ways to use Noni fruit juice included in this book into three sections. Section 1 covers different ways to drink Noni. Section 2 describes topical uses and Section 3 covers techniques for taking Noni internally.

Each chapter is also divided into three parts. In the first

part, I suggest some conditions that might be helped by the Noni application the chapter describes. This list is a guideline and is not meant to provide medical advice or to be used as a prescription. If you have a condition that is not listed, but think the application might help, by all means try it. Of course, Noni won't always help everyone, even those whose conditions are on the list. In the second part of each chapter, I give detailed, step-by-step instructions on how to do each Noni application. Third, I offer additional information about the procedure.

At the back of this book, you'll find five appendices that attempt to address some of the questions people most often ask about Noni. Appendix A, How to Enhance the Effects of Noni, lists procedures you can do to get the best and most from Noni. Several of these procedures are new to this latest edition. Appendix B lists Ways to Warm Noni for More Comfortable Topical Applications. Appendix C contains information about cleansing reactions. Appendix D offers ideas why Noni may not work for you. Finally, those who have found that Noni has stopped working for them may find some possible explanations in Appendix E. I am grateful to Dr. Ralph Heinicke for offering additional insights into this topic.

As you read this book, keep in mind that I am not a physician. The ideas that I offer for using Noni are not meant to replace your doctor's advice. I simply want to share what I know about Noni, and how my family and others have used Noni, so that you can have the opportunity to benefit as we have from this unique and amazing fruit.

# A GIFT OF GRACE:

Throughout this book, I refer to Noni's "beneficial compounds." I do not believe that Noni itself heals. Health, and being healed of something, is a gift of Grace. Therapies and supplements, including Noni, simply give the body what it needs to receive these gifts. The applications in this book can help your body obtain all the blessings it can with the help of Noni.

Best wishes on your journey to greater health and well-being!

Sincerely,
Isa Navarre

P.S. If you are new to Noni or to my "Ways to Use Noni" books, a warm welcome to you! I hope this book will give you assurance that Noni is a versatile liquid nutritional supplement and confidence to use it freely. To those who are already familiar with my books, a sincere welcome back.

# -SECTION 1-

# DRINKING APPLICATIONS

Unlike juice beverages that we drink by the glassful, Noni fruit juice servings are measured by the ounce, which equals only two tablespoonfuls. How much Noni is right for you depends on your health condition and the unique way your body responds to Noni. Several chapters in this book can help you choose how much Noni you might need (a list of these chapters is given on page 5).

Section 1 offers a variety of techniques for drinking Noni. You'll find ways to objectively and subjectively evaluate how well Noni is working for you (see Chapters 3, 4, 5 and 6). Of interest to many people is how they can use Noni most economically. Over twenty-five ways to enhance the effects of Noni are listed in Appendix A (page 397).

Section 1 also includes protocols for special situations (like trauma, insomnia and addictions), for improving your health (such as fasting, hydrating your body and improving athletic performance) and for assisting you through the trials of daily living (like sick days, family needs and stress relief). The Table of Contents will give you the best overview of what you can find in Section 1.

To get the best from this book, choose one health challenge to focus on first. Choose the procedure for drinking Noni that best suits that challenge. Then refer to Appendix A to find ways you can enhance the procedure you've chosen. Also try the topical and internal Noni applications that are appropriate for your condition. Continue with these applications and procedures for at least three months. If you have several health challenges other than the one you've initially chosen, they should improve as a side-benefit.

I am often asked how long it could take to notice beneficial effects from Noni. Some people recognize health improvement almost immediately. A few must continue to take Noni for months before they enjoy significant results. But most people will notice a difference within a few weeks. How much time your body will need to make the changes you want depends on many things. These factors include how serious your condition is and how long you've had it; what other circumstances, stresses or issues you are also dealing with; and what other therapies and supplements you may also be using. Noni might even enhance the benefits of these other therapies and supplements.

## INTRODUCING NONI DILUTIONS:

Noni fruit juice contains many scientifically documented beneficial compounds. It also contains "restorative energies." When you drink Noni you benefit from Noni's beneficial compounds, as well as its restorative energies.

Restorative energy may not yet be measurable with instruments, but it is palpable and very real to people who are sensitive to such things. Every medicinal herb and supplement also has restorative energy, but that of Noni is particularly versatile because you can isolate each of Noni's restorative energies using a different ratio of Noni and water—I call these ratios "dilutions." Several chapters in Section 1 (as well as Section 2), suggest using certain Noni Dilutions. I included them in this book because I believe the restorative energies of Noni are an authentic and noteworthy aspect of Noni's nutritional benefits, and I wanted this book to include the best I can give you from my personal Noni experience. It is okay if you are skeptical about the Noni Dilutions and Noni restorative energy. In chapters where dilutions are suggested, the added water is necessary for a logical reason anyway. But if you mix the Noni and water together as suggested, the Noni restorative energy will come forth. This will give you an added benefit.

# –1–
# Is Noni Right for Me?

Let's begin by helping you decide if you should take Noni.

## REASONS PEOPLE ADD
## NONI TO THEIR DIET:

- To improve overall health and well being.
- To boost the immune system.
- To help the body heal after injury or surgery.
- To help support the body's natural healing processes.
- To better absorb nutrients from foods and other supplements.
- To provide certain nutrients not present in adequate amounts in food today. One such nutrient is proxeronine, which is abundant in Noni fruit juice.
- To try a natural approach to health and healing to support the conventional methods they are already using, or because these methods are not working well enough.
- To strengthen the structure of the body's enzymes, cell receptor sites and other proteins in order to help all body processes work better.
- Noni helped a friend, who recommended that they try it, too.
- They are a leader among their circle of friends, and often try new things first before recommending them to others.

# HOW TO DECIDE IF
# NONI IS RIGHT FOR YOU:

1.  Get the facts and satisfy your skepticism and curiosity by reading scientific research and testimonials on Noni.

    *   For research, look up www.noniresearch.org on the internet.
    *   For testimonials go to www.nonihealthinfo.com. There you will find information about noni, its history, and stories of how this amazing fruit has helped countless people worldwide.

2.  Consider your health challenges and the goals you believe Noni can help you achieve. Be sure to write these goals down. The chapter on How to Achieve Your Health Goals with Noni (page 29) can walk you through this important step.

3.  You won't be able to truly know if Noni is right for you unless you try some. Give Noni a three-month trial. This is a fair amount of time to notice the lasting effects Noni can have on your health.

# GUIDELINES FOR STARTING NONI:

1. Decide if you should Introduce Noni Gradually to Your Diet (page 43) or begin with a Loading Serving (page 47).

2. Then refer to the following chapters to decide how much Noni to take on a daily basis:
   • The Easy Way to Select Your Noni Serving Size (page 51).
   • The Sipping Method for Finding Your Ideal Amount (page 55).
   • The Noni Maintenance Serving (page 63).
   • Noni for Acute Conditions (page 75).
   • Noni for Chronic Conditions (page 79).
   • Noni for Serious Conditions (pages 83 and 87).
   • Noni for Life-threatening Conditions (page 91).
   • The Noni Top Serving Procedure (page 57).
   • A Noni Protocol to Quit Smoking and for Addiction Relief (page 151).

3. Select a method for evaluating the effects of Noni. This is extremely important so you can assess how well Noni has helped you at the end of your three-month trial. Choose among:
   • Noni Health Evaluation Sheets (page 17).
   • Evaluating Your Progress with Noni (page 25).
   • How to Achieve Your Health Goals with Noni (29).

4. Follow the instructions in Chapter 2, "Your First Serving," on page 7.

# MORE ABOUT DECIDING
# IF NONI IS RIGHT FOR YOU:

I believe life will take care of us as long as we are grateful for everything we have and give our best to everything we do, whether it involves career, family, health, home or hobby. Plus, we have to keep ourselves open to allow life to continue to take care of us. This means watching for opportunities to grow.

In my life, such opportunities have come in a variety of ways. For example, by following an urge to go out of my way to visit the library, I found a book that helped me expand my understanding of a problem at a crucial moment. An opportunity also came when a friend mentioned a certain healthcare provider she was seeing. It felt right for me to visit this practitioner, too, and I benefited from it very much. I also sensed an opportunity for personal healing when Noni came into my life (writing books on Noni came afterwards).

Consider how you yourself heard about Noni. Is life offering you a chance to improve your health? Not everything that comes to your attention is an opportunity for stepping forward, but if it sounds significant and if it feels right, you owe it to yourself to give it a chance.

# -2-
# Your First Serving

Your adventure with Noni begins!

## DRINK YOUR FIRST SERVING:

- When you have made a commitment to improve your health and would like to see if Noni will help you achieve your health goals.
- When you have completed the Noni Health Evaluation Sheet #1 (page 20) and the Noni Progress Chart (page 26). This will take only a few minutes and is a very important step in rating how well Noni is working for you.
- When you have read Chapter 3 on Evaluating the Immediate Effects of Noni. You might want to use the techniques described in that chapter when you take your First Serving.

## HOW TO DRINK A FIRST SERVING:

1. Turn the bottle of Noni fruit juice upside down then right side up a few times. This will mix the watery part of the juice with the pulp, which tends to settle to the bottom of the bottle.

2. Open the bottle and pour about one ounce of Noni fruit juice into a wine glass. (Since this is your first, why not celebrate by pouring it into something special?)

3. Take a sip of Noni and hold it in your mouth for a few seconds before swallowing. Do the same with the remainder of the serving.

**Equivalents Helpful to Know
For the Procedures in this Book:**

Three Teaspoons = One Tablespoon

Two Tablespoons = One Ounce

# MORE ABOUT YOUR FIRST SERVING:

Sip your First Serving slowly instead of drinking it all at once. This introduces your body to Noni's beneficial compounds and their effects in a more balanced way. Try closing your eyes while sipping your First Serving. You have taken the first step on a journey to greater health, so try to fully appreciate the moment.

To measure Noni servings I use one-ounce plastic medicine cups, also called "dosing cups." You can find them in most drug stores. You could also measure Noni with a tablespoon-size measuring spoon (two tablespoons equal one ounce). Larger servings of Noni can be measured in a glass measuring cup that lists liquid ounces. When you are measuring Noni, hold the cup at eye level to ensure an accurate measurement.

If after taking your First Serving you have an immediate, uncomfortable reaction to Noni, it may be due to allergies, a toxin release or cleansing reaction, or because your body is dehydrated.

- Allergies to Noni are very rare. But some people may be allergic to the fruit juices that may be mixed with Noni to enhance its flavor. Grape and blueberry juices are commonly added to Noni fruit juice.
- Keep in mind that what seems to be an allergic reaction may really be a cleansing reaction (page 409). If you have a buildup of toxins that are ready to be released, one serving of Noni may be just enough to invite them out.

• If your body is dehydrated, it will not be able to properly manage Noni's beneficial compounds or flush the toxins that your body may release. This can cause uncomfortable symptoms that can mimic an allergic reaction. (See "Hydrating with Noni" on page 145.)

To find out more about cleansing reactions, including how to identify them and what to do about them, please see page 409.)

Store your bottle of Noni in the refrigerator. Once opened, a Noni bottle that is kept refrigerated should remain optimally fresh for about four to six months.

# -3-
# Evaluating the Immediate Effects of Noni

Not everyone can sense Noni's effects right away. But this procedure is worth trying to see if you can. You may be surprised!

## USE THIS PROCEDURE TO:

- Gain assurance that Noni can help you.
- Discover how quickly Noni can begin to affect your body.
- Preview how and where Noni may help you first.
- Test your personal level of body awareness and sensitivity.

## HOW TO EVALUATE
## THE IMMEDIATE EFFECTS OF NONI:

1. Pour your First Serving (page 7) of Noni fruit juice.

2. Before you drink the Noni, establish some reference points that are easy to self-evaluate, such as lung capacity, visual acuity and a sense of how centered and energetic you feel. A chart is provided (page 15) for you to describe these reference points both before and after you take your First Serving.

- Take a deep breath and then exhale. Do this three times. This will give you a sense of your lung capacity and how relaxed and open your lungs are when you breathe. Do you notice any tightness in your chest when you inhale?
- Look around the room to assess the quality of your eyesight. If you wear glasses, remove them while you do this. How blurry or clear do objects appear that are both near and far away?
- Then evaluate your energy level. Are you feeling tired, energized or somewhere in between?
- Finally, look within and try to sense how centered you are. This can be interpreted as your level of stress or how connected you feel to your heart or to the core of your being.

3. Now sip about one-third of the serving, and hold the sip in your mouth for about ten to twenty seconds. Meanwhile, close your eyes and tune into any sensations you may be feeling in your body. Then swallow. Repeat with the remainder of the juice.

4. Reexamine how your body feels. Do you notice anything different?
   - Take another deep breath. Are your lungs able to take in more air or is it easier to exhale without coughing? Do you feel more enlivened after taking a deep breath? Noni fruit juice is able to improve the body's ability to receive and use oxygen. Are your sinuses more open? Noni contains compounds that act as anti-inflammatory agents.
   - Look around the room. Do objects appear less blurry; are colors more vivid? This is a common response and may be due to Noni's effect on the pineal gland

and neurotransmitter receptors. Noni fruit juice also helps the brain receive and translate information, including that which the eyes perceive.

• Do you feel more energized? Noni fruit juice can improve cellular function throughout the body.

• Do you feel more calm and centered? Many people who live stressful lives find that Noni helps them relax.

• Do you feel warmth anywhere in your body? Noni may improve circulation.

• If you have a particular health challenge, do you notice any difference in your symptoms? In this case, look for an easing of symptoms or a sense that their burden is less.

• Do you feel more integrated throughout your body? Do you feel a greater sense of connection with yourself? Noni helps the cells access information about their true purpose—information that may have become buried or obscured by disease or free radicals.

## MORE ABOUT EVALUATING THE IMMEDIATE EFFECTS OF NONI:

It may be easier to notice differences in how you feel if you follow this procedure with your First Serving. The first time you take a health-improving substance like Noni, your level of health will jump to a higher plateau—whether you notice it or not. Subsequent servings will raise your level of health more gradually.

Moreover, when you body receives Noni for the first time, it may recognize that Noni is filling a nutritional deficiency. You may feel better right away because unconsciously your body is telling you, "This feels good! Keep taking Noni. This is what I want and need!"

On the other hand, after taking Noni for a while, your body sensitivity and awareness may have improved without your realizing it. You may notice differences before and after taking a serving of Noni that you hadn't before.

Try using this procedure when you introduce Noni to others. Lead them through each step as they take their First Serving. This can be a fun way for friends to share Noni with each other. (For more about sharing Noni with others, see page 217.) When you offer a First Serving to others, it's a good opportunity to repeat the procedure for Evaluating the Immediate Effects of Noni yourself.

Changes in lung capacity, vision, energy level and sense of centeredness and calmness are reference points that are easy for most people to notice. That is why I chose them for this procedure. Feel free to customize this procedure by changing or modifying the reference points or the order in which you consider them.

Also try Evaluating the Immediate Effects of Noni after Interrupting Your Noni Regimen (see page 105). In this case, your results may be even more noticeable. Your body already knows what Noni can do for it, and after being without it during the "interruption" period, your body may crave Noni all the more.

# HOW TO USE THE CHART
# OF REFERENCE POINTS TO EVALUATE
# THE IMMEDIATE EFFECTS OF NONI:

1.  Briefly describe and evaluate the following reference points before you take your First Serving of Noni. Write down any sensations or descriptive words that come to mind. Or simply use words such as "none," "not much," "a little," "moderate," "a lot," "pretty good (or bad)," "high (or low)" or "same as usual."

2.  Take your First Serving of Noni.

3.  Again describe and evaluate the following reference points. Write down any sensations or descriptive words that come to mind. Here are some examples: "no change," "more (or less) than usual," "feels a little better (or worse)," "feels different," "seems much better" or "same as usual."

## CHART OF REFERENCE POINTS:

| Reference Point | Before your First Serving of Noni | After your First Serving of Noni |
|---|---|---|
| Tightness of lungs | | |
| Clarity of eyesight | | |
| Level of energy | | |
| Degree of stress | | |
| Quality of centeredness | | |
| Other sensations that you may be aware of: | | |

# -4-

# Noni Health
# Evaluation Sheets

It is human nature to forget we ever had certain symptoms once they go away. This questionnaire will help you remember the symptoms you have now, so you can better appreciate the difference in how you feel when they improve.

## USE THE NONI
## HEALTH EVALUATION SHEETS:

- To keep track of your health improvement with Noni.
- For a comprehensive picture of how you are doing in all areas of your health.
- To track changes in minor health concerns.
- When you have health problems in many areas of your body.

(See also Evaluating Your Progress with Noni on page 25, which charts the progress of only a few symptoms.)

## HOW TO USE THE NONI
## HEALTH EVALUATION SHEETS:

1. Complete the Health Evaluation Sheet #1 (page 20) before you start taking Noni or as soon as possible thereafter. Give thoughtful, descriptive answers. Then file Sheet #1, and don't look at it until after you have completed Sheet #2.

2.  Make some copies of Sheet #2 (pages 22 and 23).

3.  After taking Noni daily for about a month or two, complete a copy of Sheet #2.

4.  Compare your answers with what you wrote earlier on Sheet #1. Use a marking pen to highlight those answers that are significantly different.

5.  A few months later, complete another copy of Sheet #2. Compare your answers with those you gave on the Evaluation Sheets you previously completed.

## MORE ABOUT THE NONI HEALTH EVALUATION SHEETS:

From time to time, monitor your health progress by completing another copy of Sheet #2. The time interval you choose between completing copies could be as soon as two weeks or as long as a few months. Be sure to keep your copies, so you have something to look back on over the years, as well as to show others who may be interested in how Noni has helped you.

You can also use what you learn from these evaluation sheets to adjust how you are using Noni. If you find your symptoms are improving, you know Noni is working for you, and you might even try cutting back your serving size. If your symptoms improve only to a point, consider the technique for Stubborn Conditions (page 99), or the Top Serving Procedure (page 57), or simply increasing the amount of Noni that you take. See also Ways to Enhance the Effects of Noni on page 397.

# NONI HEALTH EVALUATION SHEET #1

Please think about and then comment on the state of your health in the following areas. Describe how they feel, plus any pain or other symptoms you may have there.

When I wake up in the morning _____

At bedtime_____

After eating _____

My overall stamina _____

My head _____

My eyes_____

My hearing _____

My sinuses _____

My teeth and gums _____

My neck _____

My shoulders_____

My back _____

My hips_____

My knees and ankles_____

My feet and toes _____

My libido_____

My bladder and urinary tract_____

My bowel regularity _____

My skin _____

My hands and fingers _____

My nails and cuticles _____

My joints _____

My circulation _____

My heart _____

My lungs _____

Other internal organs I have problems with _____

My menstrual cycles (or how I react to hers) _____

_____

Other areas of my body not mentioned here_____

_____

_____

My energy level _____

My stress level _____

My ability to feel calm, still and centered_____

My body weight is _____

My emotions are _____

My ability to think clearly_____

My ability to remember important things _____

I am taking Noni fruit juice for_____

I think Noni fruit juice will_____

The one thing I would like most to change about my health is

_____

# NONI HEALTH EVALUATION SHEET #2

After you have taken Noni for a while, please think about and then comment on the state of your health in the following areas. Describe how they feel, plus any pain or other symptoms you may have there.

When I wake up in the morning _____

At bedtime _____

After eating _____

My overall stamina _____

My head _____

My eyes _____

My hearing _____

My sinuses _____

My teeth and gums _____

My neck _____

My shoulders _____

My back _____

My hips _____

My knees and ankles _____

My feet and toes _____

My libido _____

My bladder and urinary tract _____

My bowel regularity _____

My skin _____

My hands and fingers _____

My nails and cuticles _____

My joints _____

My circulation_____

My heart _____

My lungs _____

Other internal organs I have problems with _____

My menstrual cycles (or how I react to hers) _____

Other areas of my body not mentioned here_____

_____

_____

My energy level _____

My stress level _____

My ability to feel calm, still and centered_____

My body weight is _____

My emotions are _____

My ability to think clearly_____

My ability to remember important things _____

I am taking Noni fruit juice for_____

I think Noni fruit juice will _____

The one thing I would like most to change about my health is

_____

# –5–

# Evaluating Your
# Progress with Noni

Here is another way to evaluate how well Noni is working for you.

## THIS CHAPTER CAN HELP YOU EVALUATE YOUR PROGRESS WITH NONI WHEN:

- You have specific health concerns for which you are drinking Noni.
- You are looking for a way to evaluate how Noni is helping you with certain symptoms.
- You want a more structured and less subjective approach to evaluating Noni than that provided by the Noni Health Evaluation Sheets in Chapter 4.

## HOW TO RATE YOUR PROGRESS WITH NONI:

1. Refer to the chart below. In the left-hand column, under "symptoms" write at least three specific problems you are having with your health. (Extra spaces are provided for additional symptoms you would like to work with either now or later.)

2. Mark on your calendar a date that is two weeks away from today when you can reevaluate your health and update this chart. Also mark a date that is one, two,

three, four and six months away, when you can update this chart once again.

3.  As you come to each of the dates marked on your calendar, rate your symptoms as much worse (MW), worse (W), same (S), better (B) or much better (MB), than they were previously.  Write down your rating on the chart.

## NONI PROGRESS CHART

| Symptoms | In two weeks | In one month | In two months | In three months | In four months | In six months |
|---|---|---|---|---|---|---|
| | | | | | | |
| | | | | | | |
| | | | | | | |
| | | | | | | |
| | | | | | | |
| | | | | | | |
| | | | | | | |
| | | | | | | |
| | | | | | | |
| | | | | | | |
| | | | | | | |
| | | | | | | |
| | | | | | | |
| | | | | | | |
| | | | | | | |
| | | | | | | |
| | | | | | | |
| | | | | | | |

# MORE ABOUT EVALUATING YOUR PROGRESS WITH NONI:

Filling out this chart will give you an accurate long-term sense of how well Noni is working for you.

It may also help to record how much Noni per day you plan to take during this six-month evaluation period. Then, as you look back on your progress each month, you can reevaluate this serving size and make any changes you think might help you.

Also, work with the information in the following chapter "How to Achieve Your Health Goals with Noni."

---

I plan to start by drinking _____ ounces of Noni a day.

# -6-

# How to Achieve
# Your Health Goals With Noni

Writing down your goals begins the process of crystallizing them into reality. This chapter will show you step-by-step how to do this, and then give you a way to evaluate your progress toward achieving these goals.

## TRY THIS TECHNIQUE WHEN:

- You want to use Noni to help you reach your health goals.
- You are ready for the responsibilities that come with greater health.
- You need help focusing on your journey to greater health.
- You want to test how well Noni is helping you reach your goals.

## HOW TO ACHIEVE
## YOUR HEALTH GOALS WITH NONI:

1. Contemplate your overall health. Think about what you would like to improve about yourself. You may refer to the symptoms you described in Chapters 4 and 5 (see the charts on pages 20, 22 and 26). Then formulate your thoughts into goals. Using positive words, write down these goals. Three Noni Goal Setting Worksheets are provided on pages 30-32 for you to do this.

2. Then write down a few ways your life would change if you achieved that goal.

3. Then read through this book to select the Noni procedures and applications that you think would best help you achieve your goals. Space is provided on the Goal Setting Worksheet to write down these procedures.

4. Make a list of other things you will do to help you achieve your goals. For example, see a healthcare specialist, modify your diet, start an exercise program or get more rest. I have provided a few examples of the Noni Goal Setting Worksheets, so you can see the scope of possible goals and how these worksheets can be used.

5. Keep track of your progress using the Noni Goal Achievement Chart (page 37).

## SAMPLE NONI
## GOAL SETTING WORKSHEET:

### SAMPLE HEALTH GOAL #1
To be able to climb the stairs without stopping for breath.

**What my life will be like when I achieve my goal:**
1. We can move the bedroom back upstairs.
2. I will be able to do the laundry, since the washing machine is in the basement.
3. I will be able to tuck the children in bed at night.

**Ways to use Noni to help me achieve my goal:**
1. The Procedure for Chronic Conditions.
2. Directing Noni with Breath and Focus (directing it to my heart and lungs).
3. The Auto-dilution.

**Other things that can help me achieve my goal:**
1. Take my supplements and prescription medications on time every day.
2. Improve my stamina with daily walking.
3. Practice going up and down the stairs every day, at my own pace.

## SAMPLE HEALTH GOAL #2
To remain calm when others get emotional.

**What my life will be like when I achieve my goal:**
1. My blood pressure will remain at healthier levels.
2. I might lose weight because I will no longer need to eat to calm my frustrations.
3. I will be a better listener, which may help me understand others' problems. I might then be able to help them instead of just reacting to them emotionally.

**Ways to use Noni to help me achieve my goal:**
1. The Anti-Stress Procedure (page 119).
2. Using Intention with Noni (page 115).
3. The Trauma Serving when I start to feel emotional (page 95).

**Other things that can help me achieve my goal:**
1. Prayer.
2. Read a self-help book that addresses this problem.
3. Practice listening with all my heart.

## SAMPLE HEALTH GOAL #3
To be able to jog one mile three times a week.

**What my life will be like when I achieve my goal:**
1. I will have a regular exercise routine.
2. My legs will be stronger and my body more firm and fit.
3. My blood pressure will be lower.

**Ways to use Noni to help me achieve my goal:**
1. The Noni Top Serving Procedure (page 57).
2. Take a serving of Noni immediately before and after exercise.
3. Daily Noni topical applications on my knees and ankles to strengthen them and prevent injury.

**Other things that can help me achieve my goal:**
1. Get my doctor's permission to jog.
2. Purchase a pair of comfortable running shoes.
3. Find out from my doctor or an exercise therapist what program to follow to achieve my goal. Make small, weekly goals and fulfill them.

Now it is your turn....

# NONI GOAL SETTING WORKSHEET #1

**My Health Goal #1:** _____

_____

_____

**What my life will be like when I achieve my goal:**

1. _____

2. _____

3. _____

**Ways to use Noni to help me achieve my goal:**

1. _____

2. _____

3. _____

**Other things that can help me achieve my goal:**

1. _____

2. _____

3. _____

# NONI GOAL SETTING WORKSHEET #2

**My Health Goal #2:**_____

_____

_____

**What my life will be like when I achieve my goal:**

    1. _____

    2. _____

    3. _____

**Ways to use Noni to help me achieve my goal:**

    1. _____

    2. _____

    3. _____

**Other things that can help me achieve my goal:**

    1. _____

    2. _____

    3. _____

# NONI GOAL SETTING WORKSHEET #3

**My Health Goal #3:**_____

_____

_____

**What my life will be like when I achieve my goal:**

1. _____

2. _____

3. _____

**Ways to use Noni to help me achieve my goal:**

1. _____

2. _____

3. _____

**Other things that can help me achieve my goal:**

1. _____

2. _____

3. _____

# MORE ABOUT ACHIEVING
# YOUR HEALTH GOALS WITH NONI:

Think carefully about your health goals and make ones you will commit to working toward.  At the same time, try not to limit the possibilities.  Consider the adage "If you reach for the moon, you'll never get to the stars."

When working towards a goal, it can be helpful to periodically rate your progress. The following Noni Goal Achievement Chart is designed to help you do that.

### How to Use the Noni Goal Achievement Chart:

1.  In the left-hand column under "Goals," briefly summarize the three goals you listed in the Noni Goal Setting Worksheets.  (Extra spaces are provided for other goals you might like to work towards either now or later on.)

2.  Mark on your calendar a date two weeks away when you can evaluate your progress toward achieving your goals. Also mark a date that is one, two, three, four and six months away, when you can update this chart once again.

3.  As you come to each of the dates marked on your calendar, rate the progress you made towards achieving your goals: made No Progress (NP), made a Little Progress (LP), made Significant Progress (SP), Goal Achieved (GA).

# NONI GOAL ACHIEVEMENT CHART

| Goals | In 2 weeks | In 1 month | In 2 months | In 3 months | In 4 months | In 6 months |
|---|---|---|---|---|---|---|
| | | | | | | |
| | | | | | | |
| | | | | | | |
| | | | | | | |
| | | | | | | |
| | | | | | | |
| | | | | | | |
| | | | | | | |

# -7-
# Sipping Noni

Noni servings can be sipped or taken all at once. Here are some insights about sipping Noni.

## TRY SIPPING FOR:

- Adding variety to your daily servings of Noni.
- Both acute and chronic conditions.
- Conditions in which swallowing is difficult.
- Dealing with pain.
- Extreme illness.
- Overcoming cravings for nicotine, alcohol, addictive substances or for certain food that you are trying to avoid.
- When you want to relax and enjoy a cup of hot Noni Tea (page 185).

## HOW TO SIP NONI FRUIT JUICE:

1. Pour your serving of Noni into a cup.
2. Drink a small quantity of the juice and hold it in your mouth for a few seconds before swallowing. Take your time when you sip Noni.
3. Repeat Step 2 until the serving is gone.

# MORE ABOUT SIPPING
# NONI FRUIT JUICE:

Instead of sipping Noni from a cup or drinking glass you can sip it through a straw. Straws are especially convenient for taking Noni when you cannot sit up. If you have trouble swallowing, have someone give you Noni with an eyedropper.

If you want to sip Noni while at work or on the road, bring your Noni in a thermos. This will keep the juice cool and fresh.

For some people, sipping Noni alleviates health problems more effectively than drinking a full serving of juice all at once, as described in the following chapter. Of course, others find that drinking a serving of Noni all at once is more helpful. Experiment to see which method works best for you.

# -8-

# Drinking Noni All at Once

"Cheers!"

## WHEN TO DRINK
## NONI ALL AT ONCE:

- For a boost of energy.
- For pain.
- For injuries.
- To help wake up in the morning.
- To jump start the body into a phase of positive change in the cycle of wellness.
- When taking the Trauma Serving (page 95).
- For emotional distress.
- To alleviate hunger pangs when you are trying to lose weight (also see pages 155 and 165).

## HOW TO DRINK
## NONI ALL AT ONCE:

1. Pour your serving of Noni.

2. Drink the entire serving quickly in several large swallows, stopping only if necessary to take a breath.

# MORE ABOUT DRINKING
# NONI ALL AT ONCE:

Drinking Noni all at once is like a wakeup call that can give you a burst of energy. It also asks your body to focus on any disharmony that may be forefront in the moment. This could include physical, emotional or even mental distress.

Quickly drinking a healthy substance, such as Noni, gives the body a gentle "shock" that can send it into the active phase of the cycle of wellness. The cycle of wellness consists of two phases: the active phase and the rest phase. In the active phase, positive changes are made. In the rest phase, the cells incorporate these changes, and the body gathers its strength for another active phase. (Interrupting Your Noni Regimen, page 105, can prompt a rest phase.)

Drinking Noni all at once is most effective if you take Noni on an empty stomach. The presence of food in the stomach can interfere with Noni's ability to send the body into the active phase of the cycle of wellness.

When taking Noni for pain, first try drinking it all at once. For subsequent servings try both sipping and drinking all at once to find out which works best for you.

Drinking a serving without stopping for breath is not as hard as it may sound. Most Noni servings are comprised of only one to three ounces of liquid. Of course, if you are unable to drink Noni all at once, then just drink it as fast as you can.

# –9–

# Gradually Introducing Noni to Your Diet

In some cases it is wise to introduce Noni to your body slowly, over time.

## WHEN TO GRADUALLY INTRODUCE NONI TO YOUR DIET:

- You have a weak or hypersensitive stomach.
- You are particularly sensitive to the effects of supplements.
- Your body is fragile in the face of change.
- You are taking prescription medications.
- You are concerned that you might be among the rare few who are allergic to Noni or the fruit juices that may be mixed with it to enhance its flavor. Grape and blueberry juices are commonly added to Noni.
- You have heavy metal poisoning or severe toxicity and are concerned that Noni might detoxify you too quickly (see also the Noni Gentle Detoxification Program on page 181).
- You are concerned about having a cleansing reaction.
- You have an intuitive feeling that your body is going to be sensitive to Noni.

## YOU MAY PREFER TO START WITH THIS PROCEDURE IF YOU HAVE:

- Chemical poisoning.
- Conditions resulting from dehydration (see also Hydrating with Noni on page 145).
- Diabetes.
- Mercury poisoning.
- Parasites, causing debilitation.
- Systemic yeast infection.

## HOW TO GRADUALLY INTRODUCE NONI TO YOUR DIET:

1. Start by taking one-quarter teaspoonful of Noni two or three times a day. Drink your servings at least four to six hours apart so your body has ample time to assimilate Noni's beneficial compounds. For example, you could take one serving in the morning and one in the afternoon or evening. When introducing Noni to your diet, feel free to drink your noni with a meal or shortly after eating. The presence of food in the stomach will slow down the introduction of the beneficial compounds into your body.

2. After a week (or longer if you prefer), increase your serving size to one-half teaspoonful.

3. After another week (or longer) increase your serving size to one teaspoonful.

4. Continue to increase your servings by one-half teaspoonful every week or two until you are taking a Maintenance Serving of one ounce a day. (One ounce equals six teaspoonfuls.)

**Optional:** Measure your Noni serving and pour it into a drinking glass. Fill the glass with purified, spring or untreated well water. Sip the serving, taking as much time as you need to finish it. Or, try taking adding your servings to tea or other beverages.

## MORE ABOUT GRADUALLY INTRODUCING NONI TO YOUR DIET:

Feel free to increase your servings sooner than every week if you are feeling comfortable with Noni. If necessary, cut back to a lower serving.

You may continue to slowly increase your serving size to the levels suggested in other chapters, for example, A Noni Procedure for Chronic Conditions on page 79.

When you are measuring Noni into a relatively small, quarter- or half-teaspoon measuring spoon, hold the spoon over a clean, empty drinking glass. This way if you accidentally overfill the spoon, the extra Noni will spill into the glass and you can easily return it to the bottle.

This procedure starts with very small amounts of Noni in order to avoid unnecessary cleansing reactions. At the same time, we want to get the body accustomed to Noni's beneficial compounds, and strengthen it—slowly and gradually—so it can withstand a natural and balanced release of toxins. A Noni-nourished body is not a satisfying host to yeast and parasites, and these organisms will begin to die off. Dead yeast and parasites are extremely toxic to the body. Drinking your servings with water will help flush these toxins from your system.

Drinking a small amount of Noni in a glass of water seems to make the water more bio-available to the cells. Dehydrated cells, ironically, often resist water. Noni added to water encourages dehydrated cells to drink.

If you are concerned about an allergy to Noni, prepare a Noni

Mini-compress (see page 313). Wear the compress for a few hours, checking your skin often for a rash. If none develops, you should feel more confident about Gradually Introducing Noni to Your Diet.

## NONI AND DIABETES:

Diabetics may want to follow this procedure if they are taking insulin and are concerned that Noni will improve their blood sugar levels too quickly. However you could also start with a Maintenance Serving (page 63) or the Procedure for Chronic Conditions (page 79) as long as you check your blood sugar level frequently and modify your insulin dosages accordingly. (For more about Noni and diabetes, see page 66.)

## TAKING NONI WITH
## PRESCRIPTION MEDICATIONS:

You should be able to take Noni along with prescription medications without problem. After all, Noni is simply a fruit juice. However, Noni has also been found to enhance the effects of medications, so less medication may be needed.[10] There is no way to know to what degree Noni might improve your body's response to medications, if at all. Understandably, doctors tend to be very concerned about the possible influence of supplements on medicines. Therefore, it would be better to take your Noni and your medications at different times during the day.

Follow this procedure to Gradually Introduce Noni to Your Diet, and report any significant changes in your condition to your doctor right away (including the positive ones). Stop drinking Noni if necessary. However, your confidence and comfort taking Noni should increase with each serving you drink, especially if you start to feel better.

---

[10] Notes taken during a Question and Answer period featuring Dr. Ralph Heinicke, at a noni conference, August 12, 1997, Las Vegas, Nevada.

# -10-

# The Noni Loading Serving

The Loading Serving is suggested for those who want to begin taking Noni and who are relatively healthy and planning to take a daily Maintenance Serving (page 63), or have chronic conditions and plan to follow with the Procedure for Chronic Conditions (page 79).

## TRY THE LOADING SERVING TO:

- Relieve an array of nutritional deficiencies that you may have, which would take much longer to alleviate with only a Maintenance Serving.
- Saturate your body with Noni beneficial compounds in order to maximize the benefits of subsequent servings.
- Test how well Noni will help you clear minor health conditions and alleviate the symptoms of relatively mild chronic conditions.

## HOW TO TAKE THE LOADING SERVING:

To do this procedure, drink two ounces (a quarter cup) of Noni two times a day.

1. Measure two ounces and pour them into a drinking glass. Drink as is, or add some natural fruit juice (until you get accustomed to Noni's taste) or purified water. Experiment by sipping some servings and drinking others all at once, to see if either of these techniques works better for you.

2.  Take your second two-ounce serving at least four to six hours after your first. If you would like a stronger effect, try a third two-ounce serving.

3.  Follow the Loading Serving for one or two weeks. This will require about one or two bottles of Noni.

## MORE ABOUT THE LOADING SERVING:

Taking your servings several hours apart gives your body time to assimilate Noni's nutrients and beneficial compounds. You could take one serving in the morning and one in the afternoon. Avoid taking a serving in the evening if you find that taking nutritional supplements at that time keeps you awake at night. However, if you experience insomnia, sipping a serving of Noni late at night may help you fall asleep (see page 169).

In general, teenagers can take the amount of Noni suggested for adults. Children from age six to twelve could try half the suggested serving size for adults (two one-ounce servings a day). Children under age six may need only one ounce a day as a Loading Serving.

A Loading Serving allows you to alleviate any sub-clinical deficiencies that you may have in Noni's nutrients and beneficial compounds before you start a Maintenance Serving. Sometimes a deficiency in a single nutrient can lead to a host of symptoms and discomforts. The Loading Serving procedure can alleviate these symptoms or reduce them significantly.

After taking the Loading Serving for a few days, you may find that your body is adjusting well to taking four ounces and day and you would like to increase your Loading Serving for a stronger effect. In this case, take a third two-ounce serving for the remainder of your Loading Serving time period.

On the other hand, you may sense that taking four ounces a day is too much. This will be a subjective feeling but trust it.

Cut back to one or two ounces on that day. The next day, try to resume the Loading regimen. However, your body may simply be trying to tell you it has finished "loading" and it is ready for the Maintenance Procedure.

Soon after you begin taking Noni, you may notice that you feel better overall. You may have more energy and better mental focus, or certain aches and pains may abate. Enjoy your better health, for it is indeed a wonderful feeling. Keep in mind that progress towards greater health involves cycles. The peaks of each cycle may get higher as your health improves, but they are interspersed with valleys. These valleys represent adjustments your body is making to a healthier state and are sometimes associated with symptoms generally called "cleansing reactions" (see page 409). To prevent or alleviate these symptoms, be sure to drink plenty of purified water.

# -11-

# The Easy Way to Select Your Noni Serving Size

Don't let the fact that there are 101 ways to use Noni confuse or overwhelm you. Here is a straightforward way to determine how much Noni you should take.

## TRY THIS METHOD WHEN:

- You are not sure how to classify your condition: Is it acute, chronic or serious?
- You want a quick reference for serving size guidelines.

## HOW TO SELECT YOUR
## NONI SERVING SIZE USING THE EASY WAY:

1. First, answer the following questions and write your answer in the spaces provided:
   - Name your primary health challenge_____
   - Circle the word or phrase that best describes how often you experience symptoms:

     Some of the time          Almost always
     Often                     Always

   - Circle the word that best describes the intensity of your symptoms:

     Mild                      Limiting
     Annoying                  Severe

2. In the top row and left-hand column of the following chart, circle the words that you used to describe your symptoms in Step 1 above.

3. Find the box inside the chart that corresponds to the two words you have circled. It gives a suggested amount that you could try.

## THE EASY WAY CHART FOR SELECTING YOUR DAILY NONI SERVING SIZE:

| SYMPTOMS | INTENSITY | | | |
|---|---|---|---|---|
| Frequency: | Mild | Annoying | Limiting | Severe |
| Some of the time | 1 ounce | 2 ounces | 3 ounces | 5 ounces |
| Often | 2 ounces | 3 ounces | 4 ounces | 6 ounces |
| Almost always | 2 ounces | 4 ounces | 6 ounces | 8 ounces |
| Always | 3 ounces | 6 ounces | 8 ounces | 12 ounces |

## MORE ABOUT THE EASY WAY TO SELECT YOUR NONI SERVING SIZE:

These guidelines are not set in stone, nor are they suggested by a physician. They are amounts I would take myself if I had symptoms that matched the frequencies and intensities I've listed in the chart. They are simply guidelines, but they give you a starting point. Feel free to modify the amounts with the aid of your healthcare provider, to suit your individual needs.

Once you have selected how many ounces of Noni you need, you may now want to know how and when to take them. Refer to Appendix A, Ways to Enhance the Effects of Noni, for ideas.

Most of these ways can accommodate any Noni serving size. Or, read through Section 1 to find procedures that call for about the same number of ounces you have chosen. There will be many to choose from. Experiment to find one that you like best and that suits your lifestyle.

# -12-

## The Sipping Method for Finding Your Ideal Amount

Here is another approach for deciding how much Noni to take. This technique allows your body to tell you exactly how much Noni it needs.

### TRY THIS METHOD WHEN:

- You want to give your body exactly the amount of Noni it needs each day.
- You are not sure whether you should start taking Noni using the Loading Serving (page 47) or by Gradually Introducing Noni to Your Diet (page 43). This method gives you elements of both these other two techniques.
- You are sensitive to your body and its needs or would like to practice developing this ability.

### HOW TO USE THE SIPPING METHOD TO FIND YOUR IDEAL AMOUNT:

1. Pour one ounce of Noni into a medicine cup. Later you can pour more Noni if necessary, but keep track of exactly how much Noni you drink.

2. Take a deep breath and tune into your body. It may help to close your eyes.

3. Take a sip of Noni. Feel its restorative energy enter your body; imagine your body filling with light. Repeat Step 3, taking each sip about five seconds apart until you get a feeling of being full or complete, or until you sense you are finished taking any more Noni for now. This is the ideal amount for your body at this time. Continue to take this amount daily until you sense you are ready to try this technique again and find a new serving size. Or, customize all your servings by doing this technique whenever you drink Noni.

## MORE ABOUT THE SIPPING METHOD TO FIND YOUR IDEAL AMOUNT:

As you do Step 3, you may naturally begin taking smaller and smaller sips. Eventually, it can seem as though you just can't take another sip. Your body may feel full and unable to hold any more Noni. Or you may feel quietly satisfied that you have had enough. If your eyes are closed, you might even get a visual image suggesting that the "cup is full," or sense an inner knowing telling you there is no more room at this time for your body to accept any more. These are a few of the ways your body may try to tell you it has taken as much Noni as it needs. Be alert to other ways your body might try to communicate.

If you drink several ounces of Noni and still do not feel "finished," stop the technique. But don't feel as though you have been unsuccessful. Maybe your body really needs that much Noni. Try again another time. The more you practice listening to your body the more adept you will become at it and the easier it will be.

On the other hand, you might get a sense of "fullness" after taking only a few sips. Trust your intuition and stop; save the remaining Noni for later. In this case it is possible that your body can only assimilate a few sips of Noni beneficial compounds at one time. If this occurs every time you try this technique, you body may be telling you that it prefers several small servings of Noni throughout the day.

# -13-

# The Noni
# Top Serving Procedure

Here is yet another way to find out how much Noni your body needs. This procedure can be helpful for most relatively healthy people, except if they have an acute condition and need relatively large amounts of Noni right away. In this case, see the Procedure for Acute Conditions on page 75.

## THE TOP SERVING PROCEDURE
## CAN BE HELPFUL FOR:

- Relatively healthy individuals who would like to improve their immune system and clear toxins in order to reach a new level of health.
- Individuals who have systemic toxicity, yeast or parasites yet have the physical constitution to handle a possibly intense cleansing.
- Athletes who want to see if Noni can help them:
   ° Enhance their performance.
   ° Fine-tune their body.
   ° Increase strength, stamina and endurance.
   ° Build extra muscle or improve the quality of the muscle tissue they already have.
   ° Take their abilities to a higher level.
- Health-care professionals who want to evaluate the potential of Noni personally before offering it to patients.

- Individuals with serious conditions who are unable to afford the amount of Noni suggested in the Procedures for Serious Conditions on pages 83 and 87. The Top Serving Procedure can help them find the minimum amount of Noni they need for maximum results.

# HOW TO DO THE TOP SERVING PROCEDURE:

Plan to keep track of how much Noni you take each day by marking the amount on a calendar.

### How to Identify Your Top Serving:

1. Before you begin, fill out a copy of the Noni Health Evaluation Sheet #2 (pages 22 and 23). Also fill out the Noni Progress Chart on page 26. You will be updating this Progress Chart every few days instead of every month. The Evaluation Sheet and Progress Chart will help you determine your Top Serving.

2. Starting today, take one ounce of Noni a day. Do this for three days.

3. Then refer to your Evaluation Sheet and Progress Chart. On your Evaluation Sheet, note any changes in your symptoms. On the Noni Progress Chart, fill in the next column by using the codes on page 26 to rate any improvement in your symptoms.

4. Increase your total daily serving size of Noni by one-half ounce (or one ounce if you want to increase your serving size more aggressively). Take this amount daily for three days. Repeat Steps 3 and 4.

5. Stop increasing your daily serving size when feedback from your Health Evaluation Sheet and Progress Chart show improvement in your health. You have now identified your Top Serving.

You can also determine that you have reached your Top Serving when:
- Your general sense of well-being or mental clarity improves.
- Your physical performance reaches a new plateau.
- Your stools are becoming loose.
- You have symptoms of a possible cleansing reaction (page 410).
- You intuitively sense that you have increased your serving size enough.

If you start to have symptoms of a cleansing reaction or sense you have increased your serving too much, go back to the serving you were taking before you last increased it. This will be your Top Serving.

**What to Do When You've Found Your Top Serving:**

1. Continue to take your Top Serving daily for a week or two.

2. Then fill out another copy of the Noni Health Evaluation Sheet #2. Compare it with the copy you filled out when you began this procedure. Also once again rate your symptom improvement on the Noni Progress Chart. What you learn from these forms will help you evaluate your health progress, the benefits of this procedure, how well this procedure worked for you and if you should repeat the procedure or try a different one.

3. Then Interrupt Your Noni Regimen (page 105) for a few days.

4. Begin drinking Noni again, choosing whichever Noni procedure you prefer. Or, repeat the Top Serving Procedure starting with Step 1 when you are ready for another cycle of active health improvement.

## MORE ABOUT THE TOP SERVING PROCEDURE:

The first time you do this procedure your top serving may be as little as two or three ounces a day. Or it may be as much as eight to twelve ounces a day. If your top serving is large, your body could have a great need for Noni's beneficial compounds. Or, if you are in optimal condition, it may take a lot of Noni to elevate your performance, bring on a cleansing reaction, or put you into a healing mode, which would improve your health even more. The next time you do this procedure, expect your top serving to be different as your body's needs can change.

It you like, you can modify this procedure by increasing your servings in smaller increments. For example, you could start the Top Serving Procedure with one tablespoonful of Noni instead of the one-ounce daily serving suggested in Step 2. Then increase your serving by only one teaspoonful each three-day period.

One way to take Noni is to continually repeat the Top Serving Procedure. Again, this procedure challenges the body to a new level of health. This may involve physical, mental and emotional growth. Growth implies change, and any changes we resist often manifest as a cleansing reaction. To align ourselves with the changes we want to make, try working with the suggestions in Chapter 6, "How to Achieve Your Health Goals with Noni" (page 29).

Another option is to do the Top Serving Procedure for health maintenance twice a year, for example, once in Spring and once in Autumn. This would support the body's natural cleansing cycles during these seasons.

If you are doing the Top Serving Procedure to evaluate Noni fruit juice, also experiment with other topical and internal Noni applications described in this book. A fair test of any health product is to take it for at least three months.

# -14-

# The Noni Maintenance Serving: The Everyday Serving for Relatively Healthy People

The Maintenance Serving is the everyday serving for relatively healthy people. However, "Maintenance Serving" is a misnomer. I believe that even the smallest amounts of Noni will do more than maintain your health. Noni can improve your health, even at "Maintenance Serving" levels.

## TAKE A MAINTENANCE SERVING WHEN:

- You are relatively healthy and have only minor health challenges or none at all.
- You know that Noni supplies important nutrients, and you just want to take enough Noni to cover your daily needs.
- You want to boost your immune system and cellular health as a preventive measure against future illness.
- Another Noni therapy has alleviated or improved a particular condition, and now it is time to reduce your serving sizes to a maintenance level.
- You are between cycles of more vigorous Noni therapy such as the Top Serving Procedure (page 57) or the Technique for Stubborn Conditions (page 99).

# HOW MUCH IS A MAINTENANCE SERVING?

- A Maintenance Serving for the average adult is one ounce of Noni fruit juice per day.
- Adults who are overweight may also take one ounce per day. They need not take extra Noni. However, if they want to use Noni to help lose weight, they should consider taking an extra tablespoonful for every 50 pounds of excess weight.
- Adults who have large frames, but who are not necessarily overweight, may try one or two ounces of Noni per day as maintenance.
- Adults who weight less than 104 pounds may try a Maintenance Serving of one tablespoonful (one-half ounce) of Noni per day.
- Athletes in training may find that a maintenance serving of three or four ounces works best for them.
- See also "Giving Noni to Children" on page 197.

# HOW TO TAKE THE NONI MAINTENANCE SERVING:

1. Decide how much Noni you should take each day using the guidelines above.

2. Measure this amount with a tablespoon or one-ounce medicine cup. Pour the serving into a drinking glass or keep it in the medicine cup.

3. Drink half the serving and save the rest for later. Put the glass or medicine cup on a plate so it is less likely to tip over, then cover with plastic wrap or a lid and store it in the refrigerator. Or, simply leave it on the kitchen counter.

4. Drink the second half of your Maintenance Serving about four to six hours later.

# MORE ABOUT THE NONI MAINTENANCE SERVING:

It is better to divide your daily Maintenance Serving in half so you take some Noni twice a day instead of all at one time. Spreading out your servings allows your body to assimilate Noni's beneficial compounds more efficiently. I suggest pouring the entire serving (and drinking only half), in order to make it easier to remember and more convenient to take the second serving. All you have to do is open the refrigerator, take out the pre-measured serving and drink.

Ideally, drink the first half of your Noni Maintenance Serving upon awakening in the morning. Take it at least a few minutes before you eat, smoke or drink anything else but water. If you are a smoker who is trying to quit, you may notice that a morning serving of Noni helps curb your cravings. [See also Chapters 35 (page 151) and 36 (page 155) for information on how to use Noni to help stop smoking.]

If necessary, prepare your serving for the following day the night before and put it beside your bed. This way, you can take your morning serving as soon as you wake up. Take your second serving sometime in the afternoon or evening.

Drinking Noni on an empty stomach allows you to obtain the best and the most from Noni's beneficial compounds. Take a serving at least fifteen minutes before a meal and at least thirty minutes after one. There are some exceptions to this guideline. If you are taking Noni to help with indigestion you may want to try taking Noni immediately before or after eating. Also, taking Noni on an empty stomach can cause discomfort in some people. This may be because Noni's cleansing effect tends to target the stomach first. This is especially true if the individual has a stomach condition, or any degree of toxicity there. For example, one morning I awoke with an undigested meal still in my stomach. My morning serving of Noni gave me an acid feeling. But this soon passed, and by the way, I didn't feel lethargic that day as I usually do after feasting on such a heavy meal the night before.

If your morning serving of Noni causes discomfort for any reason, take only a sip on following mornings. Then your afternoon serving will naturally be larger if you have pre-measured your total daily serving as suggested in this chapter.

A Maintenance Serving should supply enough Noni beneficial compounds to meet your body's daily needs. When you are stressed or ill, these needs will increase. Double or triple your Maintenance Serving on these occasions.

If you are relatively healthy, it is not always necessary to measure an exact Maintenance Serving each day. After awhile, you will develop a style for drinking Noni. Some people always measure the exact amount they want to take. Others pour into a glass an amount that seems "about right." And some people just drink a few gulps a day straight from the bottle!

After you have taken the Maintenance Serving for a few months, try Interrupting Your Noni Regimen (page 105) for a few days. Do this every three or four months. Interrupting Your Noni Regimen may improve your body's ability to receive Noni's benefits, and will keep Noni working to your best advantage.

## A NOTE TO DIABETICS:

The Maintenance Serving is ideal for diabetics because of the ability for only one or two ounces of Noni per day to lower blood sugar levels. This can happen in a relatively short period of time, so diabetics should pay extra attention to their blood sugar level while taking Noni fruit juice. Those who do not monitor their sugar level and fail to adjust their insulin intake could experience insulin shock. This is a loss of consciousness that is caused by an overdose of insulin.

Diabetics can modify the Maintenance Serving procedure by taking one tablespoonful of Noni a few minutes before each meal. Assuming a diet of three meals a day, this would amount to one-and-a-half ounces of Noni a day.

Insulin-dependent diabetics should consider taking no more than two ounces of Noni a day for the first few weeks. Again, they should monitor their blood sugar level to find out how Noni affects them. Then, if they want stronger results, they can gradually increase the amount of Noni they take to one ounce per serving (or three ounces of Noni a day).

Children with diabetes can start with one teaspoonful of Noni before each meal. Older children can try two teaspoonfuls.*

Many topical and internal Noni applications, described in Sections 2 and 3 of this book, can be helpful to address the various other symptoms common to diabetes.

---

* See also *Noni: Nature's Gift to Diabetics*, by Emily Freeman and Isa Navarre (Orem: Direct Source Publishing, 2006), phone: 1-800-748-2996.

# -15-
# Getting Comfortable
# with Noni

Some people get locked into the habit of taking only a certain number of ounces of Noni, using the same drinking procedures, every day. Such a habit can be beneficial at first. But after awhile, it can make the body so accustomed to receiving Noni in that particular way that the body fails to respond to Noni as well as it once did. This chapter shows you how your body can obtain the maximum benefit from Noni even years after you have added it to your diet.

This chapter will also guide you through taking Noni in a variety of ways. Then, if your health needs ever change, you will know how to adapt your Noni servings and Noni procedures to meet those needs.

## TRY THE IDEAS IN THIS CHAPTER WHEN:

- You have been following the Noni Maintenance Serving or another Noni procedure for a while and would like to try something different.
- The serving size that you have been taking does not seem to be giving you the same support or health benefits as it did before.
- You have suddenly been faced with new challenges, changes or stress and your budget does not allow you to add extra ounces of Noni to your diet to compensate.
- You want to develop a greater degree of comfort and confidence in taking Noni.

# HOW TO GET MORE
# COMFORTABLE WITH NONI:

**One or two days each week:**
- If you usually drink Noni undiluted try taking Noni with water as described in Chapter 33, "Enhancing Noni's Effects with Water" (page 141), or Chapter 34, "Hydrating with Noni" (page 145).
- Likewise, if you usually drink Noni with water, try taking your servings undiluted.
- If you have been taking "The Maintenance Serving" (page 63) try "The Maintenance Economy Serving." Or vice versa.
- Take a different amount of Noni than you usually do. For example, drink three or four ounces instead of one or two. On another day, try taking less. For example, if you usually take one or two ounces daily, try taking just one teaspoonful.
- Try Interrupting Your Noni Regimen (page 105).
- Sip your servings of Noni (page 39) instead of drinking them All at Once (page 41), or vice versa.
- Try taking Noni at different times of the day. This will help you discover Noni's effect on your body. It will also help you find the best time of day to take Noni for your particular needs. (See also Noni and the Chinese Body Clock on page 109.)

**Here are some ideas for various times you could try taking Noni:**
- Immediately upon awakening.
- Right before a meal.
- During a meal.
- After a meal.
- Before exercise.
- During exercise. (Sip during breaks.)

- After exercise.
- As soon as a stressful or emotionally-charged situation arises.
- When you feel like taking a nap.
- Before you reach to satisfy a craving for sugar or caffeine.
- After you have satisfied a craving for sugar or caffeine.
- Right before going to sleep at night. (Noni does help some people sleep. But if you are concerned Noni might keep you awake, don't try it before days you have to wake up early.)
- If you experience "road rage" or get stressed while driving, take a serving of Noni with you in a thermos or other small container. Drink it when you need to.
- During an argument, go to the refrigerator get the Noni bottle and take a serving.
- After an argument, try the Noni Anti-Stress Procedure (page 119) or sip Noni Tea (page 185).

**In addition:**
- Experiment with other ways to take Noni presented in this book. Every so often, try a topical or internal application of Noni you've never done before.
- Play with the Technique for Stubborn Conditions (page 99) and vary your servings daily for a week or two every couple of months.
- Try the Top Serving Procedure (page 57).
- Try other creative ways to take Noni that you might think of.
- Keep Noni a Family Friend (page 205).
- Don't be shy about experimenting with Noni—or coming up with your own ways to use it.

# MORE ABOUT GETTING COMFORTABLE WITH NONI:

The philosophy of this chapter is to pay attention to how Noni is helping you and know that you don't have to take the same serving in the same way all the time. Feel free to experiment. Remember that an attitude of creativity and flexibility and a willingness to try new things make the body more receptive to health and healing.

When it comes to taking Noni, you have freedom and control. Learn to be flexible with how you take Noni and how much you take. Try to listen to what your body tells you about its needs. Change is a constant in our lives and Noni will be there to help—especially if we can feel comfortable enough to modify the way we use Noni to meet our changing needs.

# -16-
# The Maintenance Economy Serving

With this procedure, one bottle of Noni should last twice as long.

## TRY THE MAINTENANCE ECONOMY SERVING WHEN YOU ARE RELATIVELY HEALTHY AND:

- Noni has been helping you with minor health challenges.
- You are on a tight budget and need to economize.
- Your body is dehydrated or you don't drink enough water.
- You are prone to cleansing reactions.
- You have a sensitive constitution.
- Your stomach easily gets upset.
- You tried Noni before and had an aversion to it, yet you are convinced of its beneficial effects and want to give it a second chance.

## HOW TO TAKE THE MAINTENANCE ECONOMY SERVING:

1. Divide your usual Noni Maintenance Serving in half. This is the new amount you will be taking per day.

2. Fill a glass with water. Pour in your new serving of Noni.

3. Drink this Noni-water mixture all at once or take sips throughout the day.

## MORE ABOUT THE
## MAINTENANCE ECONOMY SERVING:

Assuming your previous Maintenance Serving was one ounce a day, one bottle of Noni should now last about two months if you use it only for this procedure.

By taking less Noni fruit juice each day, you are also receiving fewer Noni beneficial compounds. Yet what you sacrifice in Noni beneficial compounds, you make up for with the health-giving attributes of water, which can help your body to better receive and use these compounds.

Of course, adding more water to your diet is not always enough. Sometimes your body simply needs Noni beneficial compounds. So try this technique for a month. Then evaluate how well it is working for you and decide if it would be better for your health to return to a higher serving size of Noni fruit juice.

To read about how water can enhance the effects of Noni, please see pages 89 and 141.

# -17-
# A Procedure for
# Acute Conditions

The serving suggestion for acute conditions is taken only for as long as the acute condition lasts, usually no more than two or three weeks. Acute conditions are short-lived, usually start quickly and can be relatively severe.

## TRY THIS PROCEDURE FOR
## ACUTE CONDITIONS, INCLUDING:

- Bladder infection.
- Broken bones.
- Bronchitis.
- Sore throat.
- Cold sores.
- Common cold.
- Cough.
- Ear infection.
- Fever.
- Flu.
- Infection.
- Injuries.
- Toothache.
- PMS.
- Rashes.
- Sinusitis.
- Yeast infection.

## HOW TO USE THE PROCEDURE
## FOR ACUTE CONDITIONS:

1.  Take a total of four to six ounces of Noni fruit juice each day.
    *   Make each individual serving one-half to one ounce.
    *   Spread your servings throughout the day.
    *   Take a serving when your symptoms are particularly bothersome.
    *   Experiment with sipping your servings (page 39) or drinking them all at once (page 41).
    *   Also experiment with drinking your servings undiluted or with water, to see if either method eases your symptoms better.
    *   Also try taking your servings in the form of Noni Tea (page 185).

2.  Use topical and internal applications of Noni (Sections 2 and 3 of this book), to address each of your symptoms directly and to support your recovery.

3.  When your symptoms abate, reduce your total daily serving size by one ounce. After a few days, again reduce your total daily serving size by one ounce. Continue to reduce your total daily serving size in this way until you have returned to your daily Maintenance Serving.

## MORE ABOUT THE PROCEDURE
## FOR ACUTE CONDITIONS:

If your acute condition is severe, or if it does not abate after two or three days, be sure to consult your doctor.

Acute Conditions include a wide range of symptoms,

locations and causes. This is why Steps 1 and 2 suggest trying various ways to take Noni, to see what works best for you.

One significant way to experiment with your servings is to drink them either undiluted or with water. When Noni is taken undiluted (meaning, straight out of the bottle), Noni is more likely to stimulate the active phase of the cycle of wellness (page 107), which can be particularly helpful for acute conditions.

Adding water will ease any symptoms that may be the result of dehydration. Dehydration is an underlying cause of many symptoms and ailments. Water also flushes toxins from your body that may be causing or exacerbating your symptoms.

As your acute condition improves, it is important to reduce your total daily serving size of Noni slowly over several days. Then your body continues to receive the support of Noni's beneficial compounds as it completes its healing. Just because your outer symptoms may have abated or gone away does not mean that your body is completely healed or infection-free. It takes time for your body's systems to regain their former level of vitality. Let Noni help you in this final phase of your acute condition too.

If you are relatively healthy and feel an acute condition coming on, try increasing your daily Maintenance Serving by one ounce. This may be enough to thwart the condition at its onset. This is also the most economical approach. However, if an acute condition starts out relatively severely, don't hesitate to take a full six ounces of Noni a day. Justify the cost involved with what you will probably save in time away from work, repeated doctor visits and over-the-counter remedies.

This procedure for Acute Conditions can also be helpful for skin conditions, as it improves the body's overall immune system. Try it for acute skin conditions such as ringworm, infections, acne, wounds, dermatitis, fungus, eczema eruptions, poison ivy, insect bites, and rashes and itchiness of all kinds. Drinking Noni helps address these conditions from the inside, bringing beneficial compounds to the area. For best results, apply Noni topically as well.

# -18-

# A Procedure for Chronic Conditions

Chronic conditions are those which last for a long time, or recur frequently.

## TRY THIS PROCEDURE FOR CONDITIONS, SUCH AS:

- Aging.
- Acid reflux disease.
- Allergies.
- Arthritis.
- Asthma.
- Bronchitis.
- Chronic fatigue.
- Degenerative diseases.
- Depression.
- Diabetes.
- Environmental Sensitivity.
- Fibromyalgia.
- High blood pressure.
- Heart conditions.
- High cholesterol.
- HIV.
- Hyperactivity and ADHD.
- Hypoglycemia.
- Infection.
- Lupus.
- Neuralgia.
- Pain.
- PMS.
- Sinusitis.
- Skin conditions.
- Yeast infection.

# HOW TO DO THE PROCEDURE
# FOR CHRONIC CONDITIONS:

1.  Start with the Loading Serving (page 47).

2.  Thereafter, take three ounces of Noni a day, preferably on an empty stomach. Spread these three ounces throughout the day. For example, take one ounce upon awakening, one in the afternoon and the other in the evening.

3.  After your symptoms improve, Interrupt Your Noni Regimen (page 105) for a few days. Then resume taking three ounces a day.

If your chronic condition has a localized area, use a topical or internal Noni application as described in Sections 2 and 3 of this book.

# MORE ABOUT THE PROCEDURE
# FOR CHRONIC CONDITIONS:

If your evening serving keeps you awake at night, take it earlier in the day. It is also acceptable to take your servings just twice instead of three times a day. Either take one and a half ounces of Noni twice a day, or take one ounce in the morning and two ounces in the afternoon. If you tend to forget to take your second serving, it is okay to take all three ounces at one time. Since you will be taking three ounces a day indefinitely, your body will be receiving a steady supply of Noni beneficial compounds, so exactly when you take them is not as important.

Chronic conditions may take awhile to improve simply because they are typically long-lasting and may be deeply rooted in your body. The Procedure for Chronic Conditions is designed to promote a slow but gradual improvement in your overall health and well-being. As a result, the underlying problem can be addressed—not just the symptoms. So plan to keep this procedure a part of your daily routine, even as your symptoms get better.

A factor that can retard the healing of chronic conditions is the body's preference for things it is accustomed to—even those things that are uncomfortable, painful or unhealthy. The body can resist change, even to a healthier state. If you think this might be the reason your chronic condition is not improving, try the Noni Anti-Stress Procedure (page 119). Doors can open for changes to occur when we are able to love and feel gratitude for our body, as well as our health condition. Everything we experience has a purpose, and some of the greatest gifts in life can occur by the circumstances that surround our ailing health and our efforts to improve it.

As an added benefit to doing the Procedure for Chronic Conditions, you may find relief from other relatively minor conditions that you might also have. Improvement in these conditions gives you a strong indication that Noni is indeed helping you, even though you may not yet have seen improvement in chronic symptoms. Keep track of all your health improvements with the Noni Health Evaluation Sheets (see page 17) and the Noni Progress Chart (page 26).

# -19-

# A Procedure
# for Serious Conditions #1

This procedure is designed for acute or chronic conditions that are considered "serious." Serious conditions disrupt a person's ability to lead a normal lifestyle. Some serious conditions may not be immediately life-threatening, but have the potential to become so.

## TRY THIS PROCEDURE
## FOR CONDITIONS SUCH AS:

- Cancer.
- Injuries.
- Those that are very painful or debilitating.
- Those listed on pages 75 and 79 which you consider serious.
- Those whose symptoms plague you daily.
- Any illness or disease that is commonly considered "serious," including infections and organ failure.
- Also, a nursing mother whose baby gets sick may use this procedure until her baby gets better. Noni's beneficial compounds pass through breastmilk to help the baby. Plus a mother may need the extra Noni to support herself through the stressful times of her child's illness.

## HOW TO DO THE PROCEDURE
## FOR SERIOUS CONDITIONS #1:

1. Drink five to eight ounces of Noni fruit juice each day. Take one ounce upon awakening in the morning, one before bed, and spread the other servings throughout the day.

2. If your condition has a localized area, refer to Sections 2 and 3 of this book to find topical or internal Noni applications that you can use.

## MORE ABOUT THE PROCEDURE
## FOR SERIOUS CONDITIONS #1:

For serious acute conditions, such as kidney or urinary tract infections and other infections, continue to follow this procedure for a week or two after your symptoms go away. Then gradually reduce your daily serving until returning to a Maintenance Serving. For serious chronic conditions, you may have to follow this procedure for many months or more, even if you start to feel better. Every six weeks, try Interrupting Your Noni Regimen (page 105) unless doing so is not appropriate for your condition.

Drinking this much Noni fruit juice may temporarily cause loose stools. Weigh this inconvenience against your body's present need for relatively large amounts of Noni. The stools will normalize once your body has completed its cleansing cycle and adjusted itself to this volume of Noni. Sometimes it can be a subjective decision as to whether your condition is serious enough to follow a Procedure for Serious Conditions, or if instead you should follow the Procedure for Chronic Conditions (page 79). If in doubt, start with a Procedure for Serious Conditions. After a few, days reevaluate your condition. If you are feeling significantly better, gradually reduce the amount of Noni you are taking each day until you are following the Procedure for Chronic Conditions. But if your health starts to slip, return immediately to the higher serving size of Noni. Next time, reduce your serving size more gradually.

# -20-

# A Procedure
# for Serious Conditions #2

Here is another way to take Noni for serious conditions.

## TRY THIS PROCEDURE FOR:

- Any condition that you might consider "serious," including those on the list on pages 75 and 79.
- Auto-immune conditions.
- Nervous-system conditions.
- When the individual is very weak.
- If dehydration is present.

## THE SERIOUS CONDITIONS PROCEDURE #2 MAY BE PREFERRED OVER PROCEDURE #1 WHEN:

- You are using Noni for conditions of the extremities, such as the hands and feet.
- You have been using the Procedure for Serious Conditions #1 and would like to try something else.
- You have more than one health problem.
- You typically drink fewer than eight glasses of water a day.
- Your condition has been difficult to diagnose.
- You would like a more economical approach to taking Noni for serious conditions. (This procedure uses less Noni than the Procedure for Serious Conditions #1.)
- You find the taste of Noni unpleasant.

# HOW TO DO THE PROCEDURE FOR SERIOUS CONDITIONS #2:

1. Measure one-half ounce (one tablespoonful) of Noni fruit juice and pour it into a large drinking glass.

2. Use a measuring cup to measure eight ounces of water.

3. Pour the water into the drinking glass. The Noni-water mixture you now have is considered one serving.

4. Drink at least eight to ten of these servings per day. You can drink more if you like.

5. Feel free to sip these servings or drink them all at once.

## MORE ABOUT THE PROCEDURE FOR SERIOUS CONDITIONS #2:

The first time you do this procedure, note the water level in your drinking glass so the next time you won't have to bother with the measuring cup. Simply fill the same glass to about the same level or higher. The amount of water you use for this technique does not have to be exact.

If you have a desire to drink other beverages while doing this procedure, feel free to do so. However, your first priority is to make sure you drink your quota of at least eight servings of this Noni-water mixture per twenty-four hour period.

Use only distilled water, spring water, purified tap water or untreated well water for this procedure. Chlorine, fluorine, and other chemicals used to treat tap water can interfere with the body's ability to absorb and use Noni's beneficial compounds.

This procedure suggests taking a total of four to five ounces of Noni fruit juice, as compared to the five to eight ounces suggested in the Procedure for Serious Conditions #1. In Procedure #2, the body should utilize the Noni beneficial compounds more effectively because of the water.

# THE BENEFITS OF TAKING NONI WITH WATER

When you drink Noni in a glass of water:

- The water transports Noni's beneficial compounds to the areas of the body that need them.
- The water helps the cells absorb the beneficial compounds they need and flush toxins and wastes.
- You can give your body Noni beneficial compounds more consistently throughout the day. This provides a kind of support that may be particularly effective with some conditions.
- Noni's beneficial compounds spread throughout the body more quickly than drinking undiluted Noni. This may be particularly helpful for conditions of the extremities, such as the hands and arms, legs and feet.

It is also wise to take Noni with water for severe illnesses, autoimmune conditions, and nervous system conditions, as well as for emotional disturbances and for excessive fears, worry, and limiting mental concepts. In these cases, the brain does its best to keep the body balanced. Drinking Noni with water helps the brain to do this.

Drinking Noni with water introduces Noni's beneficial compounds to the body gently and gradually. In contrast, the relatively high concentration of beneficial compounds in undiluted Noni can shock the cells if the body is dehydrated or weakened by illness. In this case, the brain may perceive undiluted Noni as a threat because Noni seems so strong and therefore the changes it promises must be intense, although they would also be for the better. If the brain does not think the body can handle these changes so quickly, it may initiate reactions to undiluted Noni, which can seem like cleansing or allergic reactions. The brain may also respond by sending signals to ignore Noni's beneficial compounds and refuse their entry into the cells.

When Noni is added to a glass of water, its beneficial compounds are dispersed throughout the water. As such, they are less likely to concern the brain's "gatekeeper," which is located on the tongue. These compounds are then free to uplift one's health without the brain's resistance.

# -21-
# A Procedure for
# Life-threatening Conditions

Life-threatening conditions are defined as serious illnesses, diseases or injuries that keep people bedridden and unable to, or nearly unable to, care for themselves. As with the other suggestions in this book, use this procedure in addition to protocols your doctor recommends.

## USE THIS PROCEDURE FOR:

- Extensive injuries and burns.
- Serious conditions that are not responding to other forms of treatment.
- Serious illness or disease that has been getting worse for a long time.
- Times when the doctors say there is nothing else they can do.

## HOW TO DO THE PROCEDURE
## FOR LIFE-THREATENING CONDITIONS:

1. Drink one ounce of Noni fruit juice every hour. You may stretch the interval to every two hours during sleep time. Do this for at least three days. You may be drinking as much as sixteen to twenty ounces of Noni a day.

2.  Ask someone to apply a Noni Tummy Treatment on you (pages 337 and 341). This may be especially helpful if you are physically unable to drink this much Noni.

3.  After the first three days, drink one ounce of Noni every two hours. (Every three hours during sleep time.) Do this for at least five days. You may be drinking as much as twelve ounces a day.

4.  Then drink one ounce every three hours. Do this for three to six months. You will be drinking six to eight ounces a day.

5.  Thereafter, continue to drink three to five ounces of Noni a day. At this point, try Interrupting Your Noni Regimen (page 105) for a few days every several weeks.

## MORE ABOUT THE PROCEDURE
## FOR LIFE-THREATENING CONDITIONS:

This procedure is designed to saturate the body with Noni fruit juice. This is accomplished more effectively if you take your servings regularly and spread them throughout the day. One or more servings may be taken as Noni Tea (page 185) or in a glass of water.

Steps 1 and 3 propose a minimum number of days to take the suggested dosages. Feel free to take the serving size for as many more days as necessary for your condition. It is best to reduce the amount only when you see improvement.

If you are physically unable to drink an entire ounce each time, reduce the servings and drink as much as you can. If waking up to take a serving is a problem, omit the nighttime servings, but take an extra ounce or two in the morning when you wake up.

If you are too weak to drink or sip Noni, have someone give you drops of it with an eyedropper as often as every few minutes. If you feel nauseated taking Noni, try adding some purified water to it. Or, try taking the Noni with other juices or foods, but keep to the scheduled serving times. If your condition has a localized area, refer to Sections 2 and 3 of this book to find topical or internal Noni applications that you can use there. In addition, do a Noni Tummy Treatment (pages 337 and 341), two or three times a day, to help stimulate the immune system.

If your condition gets worse after your reduce your serving size as suggested in Steps 3, 4 and 5, return immediately to the higher serving. As you start feeling better again, reduce the amount of Noni you are taking more gradually than last time.

Noni fruit juice may enhance the effect of medications, so that less medication may be needed.[11] If a physician has prescribed a particular serving size of medication for you, adjust this serving size only upon his or her recommendation. Noni may also reduce the side effects of chemotherapy and radiation.

The procedure described in this chapter involves a considerable amount of Noni fruit juice. Be sure to have enough on hand so you won't run out. If taking this much Noni makes you feel better, but then your supply runs out, your progress may be seriously set back. Interrupting Your Noni Regimen (either intentionally or due to lack of Noni) is not suggested for seriously ill people until after they have felt considerably better for several months.

Sometimes it can be a subjective decision as to whether your condition is "serious," and you should follow a Procedure for Serious Conditions, or "life-threatening" and you should follow the Procedure for Life-Threatening Conditions. If in doubt, start with the more intensive procedure. After a few days, reevaluate your condition. Cut back your daily serving size of Noni only if you are feeling significantly better. If your health starts to slip, return immediately to the higher serving size.

Although noni will, in all likelihood, never reverse a life-

---

[11] Notes taken during a Question and Answer period featuring Dr. Ralph Heinicke at a noni conference August 12, 1997, Las Vegas, Nevada

threatening condition, concerned relatives can take heart in the fact that it may at least help to ease a loved one's suffering.

# -22-

# The Noni Trauma Serving

The Trauma Serving offers a surge of beneficial compounds to help the body cope with extreme physical or emotional experiences.

## USE THE NONI TRAUMA SERVING FOR:

- Accidents and injuries.
- Any sudden and traumatic experience.
- Back spasm.
- Sudden muscle spasms and cramps.
- Broken bones and sprains.
- Easing withdrawal symptoms from drugs, coffee, nicotine and alcohol. (See also A Noni Protocol to Quit Smoking and for Addiction Relief [page 151] and Noni Techniques to Relieve Cravings and Withdrawal Symptoms [page 155].)
- Emotional trauma, such as grief, sadness, pain or anger.
- Preparing the body before surgery.
- Helping the body recover after surgery.

Note: Offer a Noni Trauma Serving as soon as possible after First Aid has been applied and you have attended to the victim's immediate needs. Give Noni orally only if the individual is awake, able to drink and not in shock.

## HOW TO TAKE A TRAUMA SERVING:

1. Measure three or four ounces (four ounces equals a half cup) of Noni fruit juice, and pour it into a drinking glass. Drink this all at once (page 41).

2. Then apply a topical application appropriate for the condition, such as a Noni Compress (page 225). See Section 2, Topical Applications of Noni, for other possible treatments.

3. Take another Trauma Serving from fifteen minutes to a few hours later. The more intense your trauma or pain, the sooner you may want to take this serving.

4. Take a third Trauma Serving per the instructions in Step 3. If you still require the support of a Trauma Serving, repeat Step 3 as many times as you require.

5. Then follow the Procedure for Acute Conditions (page 75).

## MORE ABOUT THE TRAUMA SERVING:

Drinking a Trauma Serving all at once is a wakeup call that can send the body into restoration mode. Ideally, it will also counteract some of the effects of the trauma, thus reducing the trauma's negative impact on the body. Depending on the severity of your condition, you may feel better after only one Trauma Serving. But take at least three servings to help your body with its recovery.

A Trauma Serving can reduce pain and help you feel more calm, restful and at ease. Tattered emotions may also be soothed. Healing and cell regeneration may be accelerated. Bleeding can be put under control (see Noni First Aid, page 281).

If you are very weak and cannot drink the entire Trauma Serving or have trouble swallowing, sip as much as you can as often as possible.

When preparing for surgery, there will be a period of time beforehand during which you are asked not to eat or drink anything. Take your Noni Trauma Serving just before this time period begins. After surgery, drink the Trauma Serving as soon as you are able.

Some people might find it hard to drink so much cold Noni fruit juice all at once if it is given straight from the refrigerator. If you give the first Trauma Serving immediately, you won't have time to warm it. For subsequent servings, see Ways to Warm Noni on page 405, or simply leave future servings on the kitchen counter to warm to room temperature.

# –23–

# A Technique
# for Stubborn Conditions

This procedure involves varying your daily serving size of Noni in order to challenge your cells with change and stimulate them toward greater health. Use this technique to schedule your Maintenance Servings as well as the servings suggested in the Procedures for Acute and Chronic Conditions.

If you are following a Procedure for Serious Conditions, your body may need a steady and consistent supply of Noni beneficial compounds. In this case, try this procedure only after you have been following the Procedure for Serious Conditions for at least two months and it has not yet helped your condition.

## TRY THIS TECHNIQUE WHEN:

- You have tried everything (including Noni) and a health condition stubbornly won't get better.
- Certain symptoms improve after taking Noni, but then return.
- You have been taking Noni daily for a month or two and have not achieved satisfactory results with a particular condition.
- It seems you have reached a healing plateau and cannot seem to improve beyond it.
- You are looking to add variety to your daily servings of Noni.

# HOW TO DO THE TECHNIQUE FOR STUBBORN CONDITIONS:

When following this technique, you will continue to take the same number of ounces of Noni per week. But you will vary the number of ounces that you take each day.

1.  Calculate how many ounces of Noni you usually take each week. To do this, simply multiply your daily serving size by seven.

    For example, if you usually drink two ounces of Noni a day, then you take fourteen ounces a week. (Two ounces times seven days in a week equals fourteen.)

2.  Plan ahead how many ounces of Noni you will take each day for the next week. (See the examples on the following pages.) Write on a calendar the number of ounces you plan to take each day. Try to vary the amounts as much as possible from day to day:

    *   Schedule the same serving of Noni for no more than two days in a row.
    *   One day each week, plan to take zero ounces of Noni. This would give you some of the benefits of Interrupting Your Noni Regimen (page 105). If you usually take only one ounce of Noni per day, you will have to schedule these "zero days" a few times a week.
    *   Another day each week, plan to take six to eight ounces of Noni. If you usually take only one or two ounces a day, this may mean increasing your weekly allotment of Noni. But it can be worthwhile to experiment and see for yourself the effects of taking an extra amount of Noni on one day.

3. Check your plan by adding up the number of ounces you have written down for each seven-day period. They should add up to the weekly amount you calculated in Step 1.

4. Every day refer to your calendar to find out how many ounces of Noni you plan to take that day. Take half this amount in the morning and the other half in the afternoon. (Or divide the total daily serving size into thirds and take them three times a day.)

**Note:** The daily amounts given in the following two examples are suggestions only. There are almost limitless scheduling possibilities.

## EXAMPLE #1
**Step 1:** Let's say you usually take one ounce of Noni a day. Multiply one ounce times seven days per week, and you find that you take seven ounces of Noni a week.

**Step 2:** Your proposed daily schedule could then be:
1 ounce on Monday
0 ounces on Tuesday
2 ounces on Wednesday
3 ounces on Thursday
0 ounces on Friday
0 ounces on Saturday
1 ounce on Sunday
**7 ounces total**

**Step 3:** In checking your plan, you find that these daily amounts total seven ounces.

## EXAMPLE #2

**Step 1:** Let's say you usually take two ounces of Noni a day. Multiply two ounces times seven days per week and you find that you take fourteen ounces of Noni a week.

**Step 2:** Your proposed daily schedule could then be:
  1 ounce on Monday
  5 ounces on Tuesday
  2 ounces on Wednesday
  1 ounce on Thursday
  4 ounces on Friday
  0 ounces on Saturday
  1 ounce on Sunday
  **14 ounces total**

**Step 3:** In checking your plan, you find that these daily amounts total fourteen ounces.

## EXAMPLE #3

**Step 1:** Let's say you usually take three ounces of Noni a day. Multiply three times seven days per week and you find that you take twenty-one ounces of Noni a week.

**Step 2:** Your proposed daily schedule might then be:
  3 ounces on Monday
  0 ounces on Tuesday
  5 ounces on Wednesday
  2 ounces on Thursday
  1 ounce on Friday
  8 ounces on Saturday
  2 ounces on Sunday
  **21 ounces total**

**Step 3:** In checking your plan, you find that these daily amounts total twenty-one ounces.

# MORE ABOUT THE TECHNIQUE FOR STUBBORN CONDITIONS:

Try this technique for a month. If it is helping, or you enjoy the daily variety of servings, continue to take Noni in this way.

The Technique for Stubborn Conditions is based on the principle that our bodies and our cells will become complacent if they aren't challenged or stimulated. Complacent cells gradually become less healthy and vital. Change keeps our bodies alert. Alert cells, by nature, gradually grow healthier. Varying the amount of Noni you take each day is one way to provide your cells with an environment of change. This can challenge your cells and stimulate them toward greater health.

# -24-
# Interrupting Your Noni Regimen

Noni fruit juice can be a life-long friend. But every so often it can be beneficial to stop taking Noni for short periods of time. Then, once you start taking Noni again, you may feel better than you did before.

## TRY INTERRUPTING YOUR NONI REGIMEN WHEN:

- Conditions that Noni once alleviated return.
- Noni is not helping a condition as much as you think it should.
- Your health has improved to a plateau and doesn't seem to be getting any better.
- You have been using Noni daily for a while and now it is time to give your body a rest in order to honor natural cycles of wellness.
- You want to avoid letting your body become accustomed to Noni, so you don't have to keep increasing your servings to get the same results.
- You want to evaluate how well Noni is working for you by comparing your condition when taking, then not taking, and then taking Noni once again.
- You want to stimulate your body into a healing mode.
- You want to encourage your cells to use Noni's beneficial compounds more effectively and efficiently.

- Also, pregnant mothers may consider Interrupting Their Noni Regimen for one week a month during their second and third trimesters. This would eliminate any possibility, however remote, that their baby might be born desensitized, or even allergic to, certain Noni beneficial compounds.

## HOW TO INTERRUPT YOUR NONI REGIMEN:

1. Take daily servings of Noni for at least two or three months.

2. Then stop taking Noni for two to seven days.

3. Start taking Noni again, but this time try lowering your daily serving size.

## MORE ABOUT INTERRUPTING YOUR NONI REGIMEN:

If you are relatively healthy, Interrupt Your Noni Regimen for about a week every two months. This will keep your body as receptive to Noni's beneficial compounds as possible and maximize your body's ability to use them. In general, those with health challenges might stop taking Noni for only two or three days every two or three months.

When deciding how long to Interrupt Your Noni Regimen, consider how serious your health challenges are. The more serious, the less often you should Interrupt Your Noni Regimen and for shorter periods of time. Also consider how well Noni has been helping you so far and how you feel when you don't take Noni.

Do not Interrupt Your Noni Regimen if Noni has been helping to ease serious symptoms or if you have immune deficiency conditions, diabetes or cancer. These conditions require constant support.

- In the case of immune deficiency conditions, Noni's beneficial compounds can lead the immune system on a course of steady but gradual improvement. Withdrawing this support may cause the immune system to lose too much ground on its progress toward greater health.
- With diabetes, Noni's beneficial compounds help stabilize blood sugar levels. Withdrawing Noni could cause unnecessary swings in the body's chemistry.
- In the case of cancer, pain may return and tumors that have stopped growing may start to grow back. To fight cancer, the body needs constant and aggressive action. Withdrawing Noni after it has helped to improve your condition is like asking your winning armies to retreat before the battle is completely won.

Another testimony to Noni's truly amazing properties is its ability to lead the body into the cycle of wellness. The cycle of wellness consists of alternating phases of rest and phases in which healing changes take place. Both parts of the cycle are essential to make lasting improvement in the body's health.

Interrupting Your Noni Regimen initiates a rest phase in the cycle of wellness. Reintroducing Noni back into the diet can jump-start the body into the phase where it makes positive change.

If Noni doesn't seem to be helping autoimmune conditions (conditions in which the immune system is attacking the body as if it were foreign), Interrupt Your Noni Regimen for relatively short intervals of one or two days. Try this as often as every one or two weeks.  Regardless of your condition, Interrupting Your Noni Regimen on this schedule is another way to urge the body into a cycle of wellness.

Temporarily removing Noni from the diet may also prompt the cells to recognize that they cannot rely on a steady supply of Noni beneficial compounds.  They cannot become complacent and take these beneficial compounds for granted.  When Noni is reintroduced, the cells may better appreciate these beneficial compounds and use them more effectively and efficiently.

If you have been taking Noni for a while and the symptoms it once alleviated return, you may be tempted to take larger servings of Noni to maintain the same results.  Drinking larger amounts may indeed help.  But if symptoms return once again, consider Interrupting Your Noni Regimen.  In this case, the procedure may readjust the body's relationship with Noni's beneficial compounds.  It can encourage the cells to use these compounds more effectively and efficiently.  Then, smaller dosages may become helpful once again.

After you have Interrupted Your Noni Regimen, you are ready again to take a "first serving" of Noni.  Try the procedure for Evaluating the Immediate Effects of Noni.  After having taken Noni for a while already, your body sensitivity and awareness may have improved along with your health.  You may now notice differences before and after taking a First Serving of Noni that you hadn't noticed before.  The differences you notice will enhance your appreciation and understanding of how Noni is helping you.

If you have serious symptoms which Noni is helping to relieve, be careful Interrupting Your Noni Regimen.  Certainly, if your symptoms return while following this procedure, start taking Noni again immediately.  Also, be sure to alert your physician.

# -25-
# The Noni Chinese
# Body Clock Procedure

Centuries ago, the Chinese discovered that the body is sustained and maintained by an energy they call "chi." They found that chi is absorbed into the body at "acupuncture points." It is then spread throughout the body via channels called "acupuncture meridians."

The Chinese also discovered that chi moves through the meridians in cycles that follow a clock-like pattern. Each meridian has a two-hour segment in which its chi is the strongest. It is believed this is the best time to treat the organs associated with that meridian. The following method for taking Noni reflects these ancient Chinese principles.[12]

## TRY THE CHINESE BODY
## CLOCK PROCEDURE WHEN:

- You would like your servings of Noni to focus on a particular organ or organ system.
- Your health condition involves organs listed on the chart on the following page.
- You have the self-discipline to take Noni the same time each day, even if it means taking it in the middle of the night.
- You would like to try yet another way to obtain the most benefit from Noni.

---

[12] Gerber, Richard, M.D., *Vibrational Medicine*, (Santa Fe, NM: Bear & Company), 1998, pp. 186, 187

• Your body (or your budget) can handle only a certain amount of Noni each day, but your health condition warrants taking more.

This procedure can be used when taking the Noni Maintenance Serving, or when following the Procedures for Acute, Chronic or Serious conditions or other Noni drinking procedures.

## HOW TO DO THE NONI CHINESE BODY CLOCK PROCEDURE:

Before you begin, plan to reduce the total daily serving size of Noni that you usually take. For example, if you usually take three ounces a day, try taking only two. If you are following Method #2 and have chosen two organs, take one ounce for each organ. If you usually take two ounces a day and have chosen three organs to work on, try taking one-half ounce during each of the three time periods. Do not cut your total daily serving size by more than one-half, especially if Noni has been supporting a weakened condition. Pulling the support too much can needlessly stress your body's systems.

### METHOD #1

1. Study the Body Clock chart on the following page, which lists the times when certain organs and their meridians receive the most chi energy.

2. Is the organ for which you would like to take Noni present on the chart? If so, take your entire daily serving size of Noni during the time period associated with this organ.

## METHOD #2

1.  Decide which two or three organs listed on the Chinese Body Clock chart are most responsible for your health condition. You may need to ask your health-care provider for his or her input on this question. Although it may seem that we have just one ailing organ, weaknesses in other organs can contribute to our primary condition.

2.  Refer to the Body Clock chart. Write down which time periods correspond to the organs you chose in Step 1.

3.  Take a serving of Noni during each of these time periods.

## EXAMPLES:

*   Let's say you have learned that your heart condition is complicated by congested lungs. Divide your total daily serving size of Noni into two servings. Plan to take one at mid-day between 11:00 AM and 1:00 PM for the heart, and one in the middle of the night between 3:00 AM and 5:00 AM for the lungs.
*   Or, you may have two separate conditions you want to work on, such as a bladder infection and chronic indigestion. In this case, take your Noni servings during the time periods that correspond to these organs: between 3:00 PM and 5:00 PM for the bladder, and between 7:00 AM and 9:00 AM for the stomach.
*   If your problem organs have adjacent time periods, such as the gall bladder (11:00 PM-1:00 AM) and the liver (1:00 AM-3:00 AM), you could take your full serving of Noni on the cusp between the two. In this case, at 1:00 AM.

## THE CHINESE BODY CLOCK:

| Organ | Time Period |
|---|---|
| Small Intestine | 1:00 PM – 3:00 PM |
| Bladder | 3:00 PM – 5:00 PM |
| Kidney/Adrenals | 5:00 PM – 7:00 PM |
| Circulation/Sex | 7:00 PM – 9:00 PM |
| Triple Warmer | 9:00 PM – 11:00 PM |
| Gall Bladder | 11:00 PM – 1:00 AM |
| Liver | 1:00 AM – 3:00 AM |
| Lung | 3:00 AM – 5:00 AM |
| Large Intestine | 5:00 AM – 7:00 AM |
| Stomach | 7:00 AM – 9:00 AM |
| Spleen/Pancreas/Immune System | 9:00 AM – 11:00 AM |
| Heart | 11:00 AM – 1:00 PM |

# MORE ABOUT THE NONI
# CHINESE BODY CLOCK PROCEDURE:

This procedure marries certain Chinese medicine principles with taking Noni. Those who try this procedure may find that their body needs less Noni overall, and that the Noni they do take gives them better and more lasting results. This is because taking healthful supplements like Noni at certain times of the day can more strongly affect certain organs.

What if the organ you want to work on has a corresponding time period late at night when you are usually fast asleep, and waking up is difficult and if you do wake up, falling back to sleep is even harder? In this case, this procedure may not be the best one for you. But consider giving it a try, at least for a few nights, to see how well it works for you. Set your alarm or make an agreement with yourself to wake up (perhaps to go to the bathroom), during that time. Sometimes breaking a habit, routine or concept (in this case about sleep patterns), loosens our mindset enough to accept change, which can include healing.

If you find you are unable to take a serving of Noni in the middle of the night, the second best thing to do is to take a serving during the time period twelve hours away.

It also helps to take your servings at exactly the same time (within the chosen time period), each day.

The "triple warmer system" on the Chinese Body Clock chart may be unfamiliar to you. The triple warmer regulates the body's fluids, temperature, and energy through respiration, digestion and excretion.

There is another reason that taking supplements according to the Chinese Body Clock can be effective. Each time you take a serving at a certain time you are knowingly taking it for a particular condition. This is using Intention, which can be a powerful tool no matter what Noni procedure you are doing. Simply, each time you take a serving of Noni, remind yourself that the serving is going to help your body heal a specific condition. Also think about how you would like your condition to improve. Imagine living a life completely free of the condition. Read more about Using Intention with Noni in the following chapter.

# -26-

# Using Intention with Noni

Intention is the reason behind your actions and can become a motivating force for manifesting the health you want. This powerful technique can be used to enhance any other procedure in this book.

## USE INTENTION WITH NONI:

- Every time you drink a serving of Noni.
- When you are ordering more Noni.
- When you receive your order.
- From time to time during the day when you reflect upon your health.

## HOW TO USE INTENTION WITH NONI:

1. Carefully consider the primary reason you are taking Noni.

2. No matter how sick or diseased your body may be, form this reason into a positively stated sentence that reflects how you would like your condition to be, as though it were already that way in the present moment. For example:
   - I am drinking Noni to keep my immune system healthy and strong.
   - I am drinking Noni to keep my joints flexible and free.

- I am drinking Noni to keep my body chemistry balanced.
- I am drinking Noni to keep my lungs open and clear.
- I am drinking Noni to keep me energetic and mentally alert.

I am drinking Noni to: _____

_____

However, there is a way to focus your Intention and make it more powerful. Simply, abbreviate your Intention. For example:

- My immune system is healthy and strong.
- My joints are flexible and free.
- My body chemistry is balanced.
- My lungs are open and clear. I can breathe easily.
- I am energetic and mentally alert whenever I need to be.

My abbreviated Intention: _____

_____

3. Write down your Intention on a separate piece of paper and tape it to the Noni bottle. This will help you remember to repeat your Intention each time you drink your Noni.

You can also use Intention when you use Noni for an acute condition. For example:

- I am drinking Noni to help my body heal this wound. (My skin is healthy and whole.)
- I am drinking Noni now to help me fall asleep. (I am asleep. I will sleep deeply. It will be a healing, regenerating sleep.)
- I am drinking Noni to help me digest this meal. (My food is digesting. My body absorbs all the nutrients it needs.)

# MORE ABOUT USING INTENTION WITH NONI:

Write your Intention several times a day. Write it over and over again, with your heart open as though you were writing a love letter. This will help to convince your mind, your heart, and all the other aspects of your being of the reality you want to create. It also sends a positive message to the healing forces in the universe, to the restorative energies in your body and to the cells and molecules within you.

Imagination is also an important part of successful Intention. Change starts with the idea that something can be different. Manifestation begins with a thought that such a thing can be. If you want a healthy body, imagine the possibility is real. Imagine living a life completely free of the condition. Chapter 6, "How to Achieve your Health Goals with Noni" (page 29), can guide you through this.

Intention also employs the principle that what you intend shall come to pass if you believe it already has. This principle is referred to in the Bible, Mark 11:24, "Therefore I tell you, all things whatever you pray and ask for, believe that you have received them, and you shall have them." Those familiar with Eastern teachings will recognize this as employing the "as if" principle. American philosopher William James put it this way, "If you want a quality, act as if you already had it."

You can also shape an Intention from a spiritual perspective that would include all. To do this, find the highest, most positive reason you are taking Noni. For me, this reason is: I take Noni because I love God and I love my body, which is God's gift to me.

Of course, if we take Noni without using Intention, we can benefit quite well from Noni's beneficial compounds. If we use Intention, we access the powers of creation and manifestation, and our journey to health takes on new meaning, depth and possibility.

# -27-

# The Noni
# Anti-Stress Procedure

This procedure incorporates many elements of good health, including relaxation, deep breathing, meditation, creative visualization, "letting go," exercising gratitude and drinking Noni. Together, they elevate the "plain old daily serving" into a powerful health regimen.

## TRY THE ANTI-STRESS PROCEDURE WHEN:

- You are suddenly faced with unusual stress.
- You have been experiencing ongoing stress and finally realize how much you need to relax before the effects of the stress damage your health.
- You have been taking Noni for a while and would like a stronger effect without necessarily having to take more Noni.
- You would like to receive a greater benefit from any procedure for taking Noni that you may be following (including the Procedures for Acute and Chronic Conditions, and others).
- You would like to try a new approach to using Noni for health maintenance and improvement.

# HOW TO FOLLOW
# THE NONI ANTI-STRESS PROCEDURE:

Find ten minutes in your daily schedule when you can routinely take your Noni. Ideally, it should be the same time every day and a time when the house is quiet and you can be alone. If you cannot fit an extra ten minutes into your daily routine, then grab whatever time you can spare.

1. Measure the amount of Noni that you want to take and pour it into a glass. Or, make a serving of Noni Tea (page 185).

2. Find a comfortable place to sit and bring your Noni with you.

3. Close your eyes, relax and take three long, deep breaths. Let your worries slip away on each exhale. Breathe in new life and vitality on each inhale. Try to visualize stress and tension leaving your body when you exhale and youthful energy entering your body when you inhale.

4. Open your eyes and take a sip of Noni. Hold the sip in your mouth and swallow when you need to. While holding the sip in your mouth, nurture a feeling of sincere appreciation for your body, for your health and for the circumstances that lead you to finding Noni. Take your time and try not to hurry. Focus on positive thoughts about yourself and your healing, and don't let your mind wander to stressful or negative thoughts.

5. Repeat Steps 3 and 4 until your serving is finished.

## MORE ABOUT THE
## NONI ANTI-STRESS PROCEDURE:

Nurturing gratitude and love for yourself and your body, as suggested in Step 4, is another powerful way to rejuvenate and reduce stress. Try to give attention to each part of your body and feel grateful for it. If certain parts are not working as they should, send them restorative energy by feeling love and appreciation for them. To magnify the effects of this technique, touch or gently massage the parts of your body that are receiving your loving attention. Contemplate how your health condition is helping you. Are you becoming more compassionate toward others who suffer? Are you learning more about patience, or becoming more aware of how to take care of your overall health? In what other ways is your health condition a hidden blessing in your life?

The method for taking Noni outlined in this chapter can be used along with any other procedure for taking Noni. It may be especially helpful for those with serious conditions or ailments where the organs involved can be pinpointed. Then, in Step 4, you can focus love and gratitude on that particular organ.

If you are following the Maintenance Serving and taking Noni twice a day, you could combine both servings into one when you follow this procedure. If your condition requires that you take more than one serving a day, follow this procedure with one serving and take the others as you normally would. Of course, if you have the time, you can do the Anti-Stress Procedure with all your servings.

If you enjoy the effects of the Anti-Stress Procedure but don't always have the time to do it, try The Busy Person's Way to Enhance their Daily Serving on page 127.

# -28-

# Directing Noni
# with Breath and Focus

This technique directs Noni's beneficial compounds to the area of the body you want them to go.

## TRY THIS TECHNIQUE:

- To enhance the effects of Noni.
- When other Noni procedures haven't given you the results you were hoping to achieve.
- To become more sensitive to your body and to the restorative energies of Noni.
- When you can identify a particular area of your body directly associated with your health condition.

## HOW TO DIRECT NONI
## WITH BREATH AND FOCUS:

1. Pour a serving of Noni fruit juice and bring it with you to the bed or easy chair where you can relax while doing this technique.

2. Decide where in your body you would like to focus the effects of Noni. Let's call this the "target area."

3. Rub the palms of your hands together briskly for about ten seconds. Place your hands, palms down, over the target area. If possible, use both hands and put one hand on top of the other.

4. Imagine the target area to be like a pair of lungs. Take three breaths, focusing your breath into your hands. As you inhale, imagine the target area expanding; as you exhale, sense the target area relax. This may take some practice, but it is easier than it might sound.

5. Drink a sip of Noni and hold it in your mouth. Put your hands back on the target area and repeat Step 4. Swallow.

6. Repeat Step 5 until your serving is finished.

## MORE ABOUT DIRECTING NONI WITH BREATH AND FOCUS:

This technique is helpful for conditions that have a specific area associated with them. For example, for disease in the heart, liver or lungs, your target area would be these organs. For diabetes it would be the pancreas; for constipation it would be the bowels. For arthritis, it would be an ailing joint. For low energy, you would place your hands over the "dantien," an important energy center that is located on the midline of your body just below your belly button. For insomnia, place your hands on your lower abdomen. For emotional issues, or diseases that have strong emotions attached to them, try using the heart chakra as a target area. The heart chakra is another important energy center in the body and is located on your sternum in the middle of your chest. For immune system support you could use the thymus as a target area; the thymus is located behind the top of the upper sternum.

During this procedure, Noni's beneficial compounds are directed to the target area in four ways: attention, intention, the breathing technique, and the activated biomagnetism of your palms.

**Attention:** Energy follows attention. You give attention to the target area by placing your palms on it and breathing into it. Your mind then builds a pathway to that area which directs restorative energies to go there.

**Intention:** In this technique your intention to focus restorative energy on a target area is stated by choosing the target area, holding your hands over it, breathing deeply into it and also drinking Noni. The body responds by directing its restorative energies and Noni's beneficial compounds to that target area. You can enhance the effects of intention by stating the outcome of the procedure. For example, "My (name your target area) will now be stronger and healthier." Use positive words when forming an intention. You can also use the techniques in Chapter 26, "Using Intention with Noni" on page 115.

**Breathing:** The extra oxygen that you inhale when you pay attention to your breathing reaches more cells and penetrates more deeply into them. Substances like Noni beneficial compounds, naturally follow the path of oxygen into the cells. The more you practice breathing into your target area as though it is a pair of lungs, the more effectively you will be able to direct nutrients, beneficial compounds, and restorative energies there.

**Biomagnetism:** Rubbing your palms together activates the biomagnetism in your hands. You can feel this biomagnetism if you rub your palms together and then hold them an inch or two apart from each other. You should then feel a cushion of air between them. When your hands are biomagnetically activated and then placed on the body, restorative energy is naturally drawn to the placement area. Noni's beneficial compounds will be drawn there too.

If you are unsure about your success with any one of these four ways, the other three can still make this procedure very effective.

When you place your palms over the target area it doesn't matter which hand is on top of the other. Place your hands as it feels natural to you.

This technique is a good one to do before going to bed or taking a nap because it is relaxing and eases stress. The healing processes you have initiated during this procedure are more likely to continue if you rest afterwards than if you resume daily activities.

While doing this technique, you may notice tingling sensations and a movement of energy. This is normal.

# -29-

# The Busy Person's Way to Enhance their Daily Serving

This technique is perfect for those who run busy lives, as it takes little time and offers big benefits.

## TRY THIS TECHNIQUE WHEN:

- You want to enhance the effects of Noni.
- You have little time to try other Noni-enhancing procedures.

## HOW BUSY PEOPLE
## CAN ENHANCE THEIR DAILY SERVING:

To do this procedure you will be taking three deep breaths. Expand your lungs as much as possible on the inhale, and on the exhale relax your shoulders and try to empty the air from your lungs as completely as you can.

1. Take one deep breath as you retrieve the Noni bottle from the refrigerator.

2. Take a second deep breath as you pour your daily serving of Noni.

3. Drink your serving all at once (after all, you're busy and you're probably in a hurry).

4. Take a third deep breath, and then return the Noni bottle to the refrigerator.

## MORE ABOUT HOW BUSY PEOPLE CAN ENHANCE THEIR DAILY SERVING:

When we breathe, oxygen fills our lungs and is carried by the bloodstream to every cell. Noni's beneficial compounds follow the pathways paved by the oxygen molecules. When we breathe deeply more oxygen is brought into the body. This extra oxygen reaches more cells and more deeply into the cells than with regular breathing. As Noni follows oxygen's pathways, its beneficial compounds are also able to reach more deeply into more cells. The extra oxygen may also enhance the effects of Noni's beneficial compounds.

If you can spare the time, take these three breaths while standing at the kitchen counter, or sitting at the kitchen table, just before you are about to take your Noni. Close your eyes, feel gratitude, focus on feeling centered and relaxed, and nurture the roots of joy and happiness inside you. All this can be done in only a few extra seconds, but it can make a big difference in your day.

See also The Scent of Noni on page 379, which also offers a quick way to enhance the effects of your "Busy Person's" daily serving.

# -30-
## Locating Noni's Target

Healthful substances like Noni rarely work on the entire body at once. Rather, areas of greatest need or priority are targeted first. Knowing where these areas are provides invaluable information about your body as well as how to proceed on your healing journey.

This technique is based on the fact that health supplements like Noni not only have beneficial compounds measurable in a laboratory, but also a nonmeasurable but often palpable and identifiable "restorative energy." This restorative energy starts working on the body almost immediately after Noni is placed in the mouth (or when applied topically). The restorative energy of a powerful substance such as Noni can be strong enough to feel, even by the average individual with no apparent abilities to sense such things. Some people can even visually perceive where the Noni restorative energy is going when they look at someone who is holding Noni in their mouth, or who has just swallowed a serving.

### USE THIS PROCEDURE TO:

- Find out where in your body Noni might be working.
- Locate areas of your body most in need of therapeutic attention.
- Develop your personal level of body awareness and sensitivity.

# HOW TO LOCATE NONI'S TARGET:

This technique can be done no matter how many ounces of Noni you take each day.

1. Pour a serving of Noni.

2. Take a large sip and hold it in your mouth for the entire procedure.

3. Close your eyes. Take a deep breath to relax and tune into yourself.

4. Now try to sense where Noni's restorative energy is pooling and where positive change is taking place. This will be Noni's target.
   - Does a certain part of your body catch your attention right away? Does it "light up" for you? Trust your intuitive sense of knowing.
   - Scan your body with your attention. Do you sense warmth or tingling anywhere?
   - Can you sense if Noni's restorative energy is collecting somewhere?
   - If you have symptoms in a particular area, do they feel any different?
   - Look for areas of your body that feel more relaxed or that seem to be letting go of tension.
   - Does any part of your body feel lighter?

5. Continue this technique for about twenty to thirty seconds. In the meantime, swallow if you have to, but try to keep as much Noni in your mouth as possible.

6. Write down one or two areas where you think the Noni may be targeting.

**Note:** Try not to pay attention to the taste or the sensation of Noni's presence in your mouth. Do your best to tune into other parts of your body. If the taste is too distracting, mix the Noni with some water and try again.

## MORE ABOUT LOCATING NONI'S TARGET:

When you are finished with the technique, swallow the Noni unless you have mercury poisoning in your mouth, amalgam fillings, cancer in your head or mouth, or a serious mouth or gum infection. In these cases spit out the Noni because it can absorb toxins that you're better off not swallowing. (See the Oral Detox on page 371.)

This technique for Locating Noni's Target teaches body awareness and sensitivity. These skills are invaluable for they can also help you evaluate other nutritional supplements and even foods by using this same technique. Simply hold the item you want to test in your mouth, close your eyes, tune into your body and sense if the substance is good for you and where in your body it is targeting its restorative energy.

If you want to master this technique, you must practice it. Try it with at least one sip from each serving of Noni that you take each day. Results may be more apparent if you do this technique when taking your First Serving or after you have Interrupted Your Noni Regimen.

The reason I urge people to practice and find success with this technique is the wealth of information you can gain from it. For example, once when doing this technique, I noticed a tingling sensation in my wrists and forearms. At the time, I had a relatively serious health condition that had nothing to do with my wrists and forearms. So why did the restorative energy pool there? I soon realized I had been resting my wrists and forearms on the edge of my laptop computer, and likely, the electromagnetic radiation (EMR) from the laptop's strong battery was draining the vitality from those areas of my body. The restorative energy was pooling there to counteract the negative effects of the EMR. As a result of this experience, I installed a separate keyboard, which kept my body farther away from the EMR source. This of course, allowed the restorative energy to then address other, more important health issues.

# -31-
# The Auto-dilution

When you hold Noni fruit juice under the tongue, it becomes diluted with a certain amount of saliva. The resulting mixture forms an "auto-dilution," a custom-made remedy tailored to the body's current needs.

## TRY THE AUTO-DILUTION
## FOR CONDITIONS SUCH AS:

- Auto-immune diseases.
- Biochemical imbalances.
- Chronic Fatigue Syndrome.
- Cravings for addictive substances.
- Depression.
- Eating disorders.
- Emotional stress.
- Extreme fatigue.
- Grief.
- Low energy and vitality.
- Mental illness.
- Profound sadness.
- Trauma (after taking a Trauma Serving).
- Undiagnosable conditions.
- Withdrawal symptoms.

# HOW TO DO THE AUTO-DILUTION:

1.  Hold a small sip of Noni fruit juice under your tongue. To seal the Noni under your tongue, press the top of your tongue up against the roof of your mouth. Put the front of your tongue against the back of your lower front teeth. This is a natural position for your tongue.

2.  Keep the Noni under your tongue for as long as possible. Meanwhile, saliva will naturally mix with the Noni. Swallow as you need to, but continue to hold what remains of the Noni under your tongue.

3.  The procedure is over when it tastes as though there is no longer any Noni left under your tongue. This should occur within a few minutes.

# MORE ABOUT THE AUTO-DILUTION:

Use the Auto-dilution procedure as often as you like. You could even drink all of your Noni servings this way. Do the Auto-dilution at least fifteen minutes before eating or drinking, and thirty minutes before brushing your teeth.

It is easier to do the Auto-dilution when your attention is involved with something other than thinking about holding Noni under your tongue. One idea is to do the Auto-dilution while taking a shower, doing dishes or watching television. Or you could use this time to take deep breaths and utilize some of the ideas in The Noni Anti-Stress Procedure on page 119.

After taking the Auto-dilution, you may feel more centered with greater emotional calmness, and have increased energy, vitality and alertness. The Auto-dilution is the best way for someone debilitated with illness to take Noni. Use an eyedropper to place a small amount of Noni under the person's tongue.

The Auto-dilution can be used as the Noni equivalent of the homeopathic Rescue Remedy®.

If you have a serious condition located in your head or brain, take extra care to hold your tongue securely against the roof of your mouth. Do not allow the Noni to make prolonged contact with the roof of your mouth, as it can draw toxins from the head through the soft palate. See The Oral Detox Procedure on page 371.

Noni fruit juice contains many scientifically documented beneficial compounds. It also contains restorative energy. When you drink Noni, you benefit from both. Restorative energy may not yet be measurable with instruments, but it is palpable and very real to people who are sensitive to such things.

Noni's restorative energy can be directed anywhere in the body using a variety of techniques. Using Intention with Noni (page 115) and Directing Noni with Breath and Focus (page 123) are two techniques that instruct Noni's restorative energies to work on areas you choose. The Auto-dilution directs Noni's restorative energies to those places where the body knows it needs Noni, but you may not be able to consciously identify. This makes the Auto-dilution ideal for conditions that don't have a specific organ or tissue associated with them, or with conditions that are throughout the body or unable to be diagnosed.

Here's how the Auto-dilution works: A person's saliva carries the energetic signature of their physical and emotional makeup, which includes information, in the form of certain frequencies, about specific weaknesses and malfunctions. When Noni is held in prolonged contact with saliva, Noni's restorative energies highlight these deficient frequencies. Thus, the body is reminded of its weak and malfunctioning areas and sends Noni's restorative energies to them.

The dilution of Noni and saliva that each person produces is unique and special. The Auto-dilution helps to normalize body functions and return harmony to the individual. For example, if body weight is an issue and you use the Auto-dilution regularly, it may affect your appetite according to your body's needs. If Noni increases your appetite, you may be deficient in one or more nutrients. The Auto-dilution is simply telling your body to eat more in order to obtain these nutrients. Try a full-spectrum nutritional supplement and the food cravings should go away. On the other hand, the Auto-dilution may decrease your appetite if you have been eating too much or if you are physically and emotionally ready to lose some weight.

# -32-

# Taking Noni with
# Herbs and Supplements

Here is a reminder about something that may seem obvious:

## TAKE NONI WITH OTHER SUPPLEMENTS:

- As part of your daily routine.
- To get the maximum benefit from all your supplements.

## HOW TO TAKE NONI
## WITH OTHER SUPPLEMENTS:

1. Measure the serving of Noni that you want to take.

2. Gather the other supplements you want to take. These can include vitamins, minerals, herbs and antioxidants. Also fill a glass with purified water to help you take these supplements.

3. Drink your serving of Noni. Immediately afterwards, take the supplements.

## MORE ABOUT TAKING
## NONI WITH OTHER SUPPLEMENTS:

Get into the routine of taking Noni with your other supplements, and you will be less likely to forget to take either of them. I believe that healthful supplements have a synergistic effect. They help each other to be absorbed into the body, and then they help each other work for the body's benefit.

A leading international Noni fruit juice bottling company and exporter now produces a concentrated form of Noni, which they combine with other herbs. They discovered that Noni's beneficial compounds naturally complement an herb's healing properties and that Noni is an effective delivery system. This means that Noni helps herbs react more favorably to the human body. These findings suggest that Noni may be able to enhance the effectiveness of any nutritional supplement because it makes the body better prepared to receive it.

However, do not reduce the amount of supplements you take without consulting your healthcare provider. There is no way to know to what degree Noni improves your body's unique ability to absorb supplements. The excess supplements your body does not need are usually passed in the urine.

Consider the serving of Noni that you take with supplements as one of the servings of Noni that you take each day. In other words, you do not have to take extra Noni when taking it with supplements.

Use distilled water, spring water, purified tap water or untreated well water when taking your supplements. Chlorine, fluorine or other chemicals used to treat tap water can interfere with the body's ability to absorb and use Noni's beneficial compounds.

Also try adding Noni to herbal teas, herbal poultices and herbal baths. Add as much as one tablespoonful of Noni to a cup of tea. Add as much as two or three ounces of Noni to herbal poultices or baths. Use your judgment as to how much Noni to add to herbs based on the quantity of herbs used and the size of the area to be covered.

Herbal tinctures are best mixed with Noni rather than taking the two separately. Add one dropperful of herbal tincture to one ounce of Noni fruit juice. Gently stir the two liquids together to combine them. Take this serving size two to five times a day, depending on the severity of your condition.

Noni fruit juice can also be mixed with other medicinal fruit extracts such as Saw Palmetto berry extract and Hawthorne berry extract. Mix one dropperful of extract with one ounce of Noni, as described in the previous paragraph. Saw Palmetto berry extract is traditionally used for prostate conditions. By itself, Noni does not reach the prostate gland as effectively as it does when combined with Saw Palmetto, which draws Noni's beneficial compounds to that area. Hawthorne berry is traditionally used for heart conditions, and can focus Noni's beneficial compounds in the heart tissue.

Undiluted Noni can also be mixed with fresh garlic to help lower cholesterol levels—a traditional use of garlic. Both the garlic and Noni tend to make each other more potent. To try this combination: mix one clove of crushed (not chopped) garlic per ounce of Noni fruit juice. Allow the mixture to rest in the refrigerator a few hours or overnight. Strain the garlic pieces. Then drink a tablespoonful of this mixture at least once a day. If you find the taste of the Noni-garlic mixture too strong by itself, try adding it to other foods. It tastes delicious with a little olive oil, over salad.

I have also found that Noni fruit juice does not interfere with homeopathic remedies, but should be taken about fifteen minutes beforehand. Taking a homeopathic remedy after taking Noni seems to enhance the remedy's effects.

In addition, many Noni enthusiasts are having a great deal of success combining Noni with inositol, a vitamin in the B complex. They have used it to alleviate the symptoms of a variety of conditions including diabetes, multiple sclerosis, arthritis and severe nerve pain.

It is better to take Noni and prescription medications at different times. (For more information, see page 46.)

# -33-

# Enhancing Noni's
# Effects with Water

Here is a way to take Noni that should help your body accept Noni's beneficial compounds more easily and effectively.

## TRY ENHANCING NONI'S
## EFFECTS WITH WATER WHEN:

- You have been drinking Noni for a while and would like to try a new technique.
- The amount you have been taking is no longer supporting your health as effectively as it once did.
- You have health challenges that indicate taking several ounces of Noni a day, but your body (or your budget) can handle only one or two.
- You typically drink fewer than eight glasses of water a day.
- You have relatively mild symptoms of dehydration such as dry mouth, dry eyes or dry skin.
- Drinking Noni tends to upset your stomach, make you lightheaded or initiate uncomfortable cleansing reactions.
- You would like to be free of addictive substances and the cravings for them.

# HOW TO ENHANCE
# NONI'S EFFECTS WITH WATER:

Before you begin, decide how many ounces of Noni you would like to take per day (or are already taking). Multiply this number by two. The answer you get will be the number of times you should do the following procedure each day:

1. Fill an eight-ounce glass with purified water.

2. Drink the water.

3. Slowly sip one tablespoonful of Noni fruit juice, allowing the juice to remain on your tongue for a few seconds with each sip.

4. Spread your servings throughout the day.

## MORE ABOUT ENHANCING
## NONI'S EFFECTS WITH WATER:

Keep track of how many tablespoonfuls of Noni you take each day. An easy way to do this is to mark each serving on a notepad or calendar.

There are two ways this technique enhances Noni's effects: First, the body is given water to hydrate it, and second it is given undiluted Noni. Drinking a glassful of water satisfies thirsty cells and lubricates the body, allowing Noni's beneficial compounds to reach and enter the cells that need them. Then drinking undiluted Noni stimulates the body into a healing mode. This is the important difference between this technique and other Noni techniques in which Noni is mixed with water. Drinking Noni mixed with water tends to have a gentler and more widespread effect on the body.

The presence of undiluted Noni on the tongue tells the brain that a significant substance is now inside the body. The brain cannot ignore undiluted Noni. If the body is functioning as it should and is well-enough hydrated, the brain will respond by signaling which cells should receive Noni's beneficial compounds. It will also help distribute these compounds to those areas that need them.

Thus, this procedure gives you all the benefits of taking Noni undiluted, plus it gives the body the water it needs to get the most and the best from Noni's beneficial compounds. For a further comparison of taking Noni undiluted or mixed with water, please read, "More about the Noni Procedure for Serious Conditions #2," on pages 88-90.

It is amazing how much more powerful a serving of Noni can be when you precede it with a glassful of water. If you sense a cleansing reaction coming on after you do this technique, drink another glass or half-glass of water. If you are sensitive to supplements or prone to cleansing reactions, sip the Noni slowly and evaluate how you are feeling after each sip. You may not need to finish the entire tablespoon serving.

# -34-
# Hydrating with Noni

Water is essential to life and most people don't drink enough. This technique offers a system for adding enough water to your diet while getting the best and the most from Noni's beneficial compounds.

## TRY HYDRATING WITH NONI WHEN:

- You do not drink at least eight glasses of water a day.
- You have common symptoms of dehydration such as dry skin, dry eyes, chronically dry and scratchy throat, constipation and concentrated urine.
- You have other symptoms that are also now attributed to dehydration, including tiredness, irritability, anxiousness, insomnia, depression, cravings, asthma, allergies, hypertension, Type II diabetes, autoimmune diseases, heartburn, dyspeptic pain, angina, lower back pain, rheumatoid joint pains including ankylosing spondylitis, migraine headaches, colitis, fibromyalgia, bulimia and morning sickness during pregnancy.[13]
- You are addicted to legal or illegal substances. (It has been noted that addicts drink almost no water and are extremely constipated.[14])
- You have tried other methods including other Noni procedures, and you are not getting satisfactory results.

---

[13] F. Batmanghelidj, M.D., *Water for Health, for Healing, for Life: You're not Sick, You're Thirsty,* (New York: Warner Books), pp.58-60.
[14] Dr. Mona Harrison, *What Else Every Doctor Should Know: An Introduction to Noni and the Brains,* (Orem: Direct Source Publishing), 2002, p. 26

# HOW TO HYDRATE
# YOUR BODY WITH NONI:

You will need four one-quart mason jars for this procedure.

1. Decide how much Noni fruit juice to take each day. As your body becomes more hydrated, it will begin to use Noni beneficial compounds more efficiently and you may need less Noni than before.

   • If you usually take one ounce of Noni each day, continue to take one ounce.

   • If you usually take two ounces of Noni, try just one ounce.

   • If you usually take three or four ounces, try just two ounces.

   • If you usually take five or more ounces, try just four ounces.

2. Add two cups of water to a mason jar. The jar will be half-filled. Pour in your daily serving of Noni. Drink the entire amount by the end of the day. Repeat this step for three days.

3. Fill the mason jar with water (it will contain four cups). Pour in your daily serving of Noni. Drink the entire amount by the end of the day. Repeat this step for three to five days.

4. Fill one mason jar and half-fill a second mason jar with water. Measure your serving of Noni. Divide the Noni between the two jars, adding more Noni to the jar that is full of water. It doesn't matter exactly how much Noni you put in each jar. Drink the entire amount by the end of the day. Repeat this step for a week.

5. Fill two mason jars with water. Measure your daily

serving of Noni, and pour about half of it into each jar. Drink the entire amount by the end of the day. Repeat this step for a week.

Note that this amount—two quarts or eight cups—is the recommended minimum amount of water that most medical professionals suggest we drink each day.

In the follow steps, we will continue to add more water to the daily diet, so the water can act therapeutically.

6. Fill two and a half mason jars with water. Measure your daily serving of Noni and pour some into each jar. Drink the entire amount by the end of the day. Repeat this step for a week.

7. Fill three mason jars with water. Measure your daily serving of Noni and pour some into each jar. Drink the entire amount by the end of the day. Repeat this step for a week.

   **Optional:** Do the same with four mason jars of water.

8. Return to Step 5 and continue taking this amount of water for the rest of your life. Add Noni to the water, or try another procedure for taking your daily Noni servings.

## MORE ABOUT HYDRATING YOUR BODY WITH NONI:

Prepare the Noni-water mixture every morning. You can use pitchers instead of mason jars if you have them and you find them more convenient. Keep the containers covered in the refrigerator if you like cold liquids or out on the kitchen counter if you prefer liquids at room temperature. The Noni should not spoil if kept outside the refrigerator for one day.

Use distilled water, spring water, purified tap water or untreated well water. Chlorine, fluorine or other chemicals used to treat tap water can interfere with the body's ability to absorb and use Noni's beneficial compounds.

I find it better to drink the Noni-water in relatively large portions of one or two cups at a time. If you sip the Noni-water throughout the day, you will be more likely to visit the bathroom more often. Drinking larger servings helps to train your bladder to hold more liquid. This makes life a lot easier when you are drinking adequate amounts of water every day.

Do not be concerned that drinking more than the recommended daily amount of liquid will increase fluid retention. The body often retains fluid as a result of dehydration. Drinking enough water will normalize the fluid content throughout your body. In fact, one doctor states that "Water is the best natural diuretic that exists."[15]

Cells also store fat to protect themselves from toxins that a well-hydrated body would otherwise flush away. After a few days, your "water weight" should normalize and then your body can begin to let go of excess body fat, assuming you are otherwise eating sensibly. Exercise, of course, is also an essential element to health.

In addition, be sure to take supplemental calcium and potassium, which is necessary to regulate the water content in the body. Sodium also needs to be replaced as it gets flushed from our system as we drink more and pass more urine.

Hydrating the body is essential to get the best and the most from Noni's beneficial compounds. People who are dehydrated often have a natural aversion to Noni. Either it tastes or smells repulsive or they feel worse after trying a serving or two. This can occur because the brain knows the body does not have enough water to distribute Noni properly, or that Noni may flood

---

[15] F. Batmanghelidj, M.D., p. 248.

dehydrated cells with more beneficial compounds than they can handle. The brain knows that the body must satisfy its need for water first. Only then it can take full advantage of Noni's beneficial compounds.

If you typically have not been drinking enough water, it may take a few weeks before your body rehydrates enough to be able to optimally accept and respond to Noni's beneficial compounds. So try this technique for at least a month before evaluating how well Noni is helping you.

# -35-

# A Noni Protocol
# to Quit Smoking
# and for Addiction Relief

A first step.

## USE THIS PROTOCOL TO:

- Help you quit addictions to legal and illegal substances including cigarettes, alcohol, narcotics and caffeine.
- Support your body after you have quit, so you can enjoy life addiction-free.
- Help you release your need for foods that you crave but are allergic to, that suppress your health, or that prevent weight loss.

## HOW TO FOLLOW THE PROTOCOL TO QUIT SMOKING AND FOR ADDICTION RELIEF:

1. Fill an eight-ounce glass with purified, distilled or spring water.

2. Drink the water.

3. Take one ounce of Noni following each glass of water. Sip or drink the Noni all at once, as you prefer.

4. Take eight of these servings each day.

## WHEN TO DO THE ABOVE PROCEDURE:

- Put a glass of water and an ounce of Noni beside your bed each night, so you can drink the water and Noni first thing when you wake up in the morning.
- If you are not ready to quit, and hope Noni can give you the support you need to make quitting easier, spread the eight servings throughout the day.
- If you have quit, take a serving of water and Noni each time you feel a craving; otherwise spread your servings throughout the day.
- Before bed, take an extra serving of Noni or use one of the techniques in Chapter 36.
- If you have taken the eight servings and still suffer from cravings and withdrawal symptoms, drink additional servings of water and Noni if necessary. See A Noni Procedure for Life-threatening Conditions, on page 91. See also Noni Techniques to Relieve Cravings and Withdrawal Symptoms, on page 155.

## MORE ABOUT THE PROTOCOL TO QUIT SMOKING AND TO RELIEVE ADDICTIONS:

Drinking eight glasses of water a day is the minimum amount suggested by most medical professionals. The three primary reasons for drinking enough water and Noni fruit juice when you quit cigarettes or other addictive substances are to help your body normalize its metabolism, to release its physiological need for the substance, and to flush your cells of the addictive substance or toxins associated with it. These toxins will cause you to crave more of the addictive substance. For example, water flushes nicotine from the body. The less nicotine in your body, the less you will crave it.

Water also allows Noni beneficial compounds to work their best. For the benefits of drinking Noni after drinking water, please see "More about Enhancing Noni's Effects with Water" on page 141.

In addition, Dr. Mona Harrison writes, "It should be further noted that most people who are addicted to legal and illegal substances drink almost no water and are extremely constipated."[16] Return water to the diet and the cravings should diminish or go away.

If you find it difficult to drink this much water at first, start with half-glasses followed by an ounce of Noni. Gradually increase the amount of water you drink until you have reached the goal of eight full glasses a day.

When quitting cigarettes, don't be surprised if you or your family smells nicotine emanating from your body, even though you are not smoking anymore. This odor means your body is eliminating nicotine through your skin. Your body may need more Noni during the first week after your last cigarette, when the nicotine release is at its peak. Increase your serving size if necessary during this time.

Overcoming any addiction may require relatively large quantities of Noni fruit juice at first. Drink at least the suggested eight ounces of Noni a day until your cravings come under control and you are free of withdrawal symptoms. Then reduce the number of ounces you take each day until you find a serving size that allows you to enjoy life without having to suffer cravings. Continue to drink eight or more glasses of water a day.

## WHY NONI WORKS SO WELL FOR ADDICTION RELIEF:

The following is based on A.K. Olsen's interviews with Dr. Ralph Heinicke, the world's leading authority on xeronine.[17]

---

[16] Dr. Mona Harrison, *What Else Every Doctor Should Know: An Introduction to Noni and the Brains,* (Orem: Direct Source Publishing), 2002, p. 26

[17] *Understanding the Miracle: An Introduction to the Science of Noni,* A series of interviews conducted by A.K. Olsen with Dr. Ralph Heinicke, from June 1998 to August 1998 (Direct Source), p. 14.

Noni provides essential ingredients that the body needs to make xeronine. Xeronine is a type of body chemical called an "alkaloid," and it is essential for health. Nicotine is also an alkaloid. In fact, the nicotine and xeronine alkaloids are shaped very much the same. Other addictive substances such as caffeine, cocaine, heroin and morphine are also alkaloids that look very much like xeronine.

However, the body does not get "addicted" to xeronine because the body manufactures it naturally. (One cannot get addicted to Noni, either.) The explanation in the following paragraphs refers to nicotine, but it pertains to other addictive alkaloids as well.

When an individual smokes a cigarette, the brain is flooded with nicotine. Because nicotine and xeronine look so much alike, the brain cells will accept nicotine in place of xeronine simply because there is more of it. If the brain is flooded with nicotine over several days, the cell receptors will actually adjust their shape, so they prefer the nicotine alkaloids instead of xeronine alkaloids. Feedback mechanisms tell the body it can lower its production of xeronine because the addictive alkaloids are taking its place. At this point, the individual is addicted. The brain cells now have a physical need for nicotine.

However, this action can also work in reverse. If you flood the brain with xeronine (by drinking relatively large servings of Noni) and stop providing additional nicotine, then after several days the brain cell receptors will again adjust themselves. Only now they will prefer xeronine instead of nicotine, as they normally should, and the body will start producing more of its own xeronine once again. Now there is no addiction.

# -36-

## Noni Techniques to Relieve Cravings and Withdrawal Symptoms

The following techniques include several forms of Noni: Noni liquid concentrate, Noni skin lotion, Noni seed oil and Noni fruit juice.

### USE THE TECHNIQUES IN THIS CHAPTER TO:

- Alleviate withdrawal symptoms.
- Find freedom from addictions to legal or illegal substances.
- Free yourself from food cravings that lead to weight problems.
- Obtain relief from cravings for cigarettes, alcohol and other addictive substances.
- Support your body while you become addiction-free.

# TECHNIQUES TO RELIEVE CRAVINGS AND WITHDRAWAL SYMPTOMS:

**Take Noni Liquid Concentrate Orally**

1. Put two drops of Noni liquid concentrate under your tongue, one on the right side and one on the left.

2. Do this every waking hour for the first three days after you have stopped taking the addictive substance. For the next week, do it three times a day. The following week you may need to do it only once a day.

Placing Noni liquid concentrate under your tongue allows Noni's beneficial compounds to go directly to your brain. Doing this every hour ensures that the brain is kept flooded with these compounds. This essential step helps your brain cells relearn how to prefer natural xeronine instead of addictive alkaloids. (This change of preference is explained under the heading "Why Noni Works so Well for Addiction Relief," on page 154.)

The gradual reduction in amounts of Noni concentrate is meant to correspond with the decrease of addictive alkaloids in the brain.

Noni liquid concentrate is available from those who also distribute Noni fruit juice. If you are unable to obtain Noni liquid concentrate, try this technique using the Auto-dilution on page 133.

**Use Noni Liquid Concentrate Topically**

1. Put three drops of skin lotion in the palm of your hand.

2. Add one drop of Noni liquid concentrate and mix the ingredients together with a fingertip.

3.  Put about half the mixture on one temple (the flat region on either side of your forehead), and half on the other.

4.  Using your fingertips, rub both temples simultaneously in a soothing, circular motion. You may also rub some of the lotion onto your forehead. Your skin should soak up this mixture in about a minute.

This technique serves two purposes. First, it is another way to get Noni's beneficial compounds into the brain—through the temples. Second, massaging the temples and forehead can alleviate the stress and tension that often occur when letting go an addiction.

Because this lotion-concentrate mixture is a brownish color that will be evident when applied to fair skin, some people may prefer to use only a small dab of this mixture when at work or in public. Or use Noni seed oil instead.

Use any leftover mixture as hand lotion or apply it to other dry skin.

**Noni Seed Oil Remedy #1**

1.  Put one drop of Noni seed oil on a fingertip.

2.  Rub this mixture above your upper lip and on the bottom of your nostrils. Focus on the aroma if you are able to detect it (most smokers have a reduced sense of smell).

The mild aroma of Noni seed oil soothes and calms the brain and takes the edge off cravings. The midpoint between your nose and upper lip is also an energy point that, when stimulated by Noni seed oil, helps balance the left and right sides of the brain. This can help your cells adapt themselves to being free of addictive alkaloids.

**Noni Seed Oil Remedy #2**
1. Tear a cotton ball in half.

2. Put a few drops of Noni seed oil on the cotton.

3. Dab the oil on the point above the center of your upper lip, at the base of your nostrils. Inhale through your nose to breathe in the scent of Noni. Lower your hand that is holding the cotton ball.

4. Repeat Step 3 at least ten times. No need to breath deeply each time.

This technique allows your hand and arm to follow an ingrained pattern—that of moving towards your mouth. But rather than making this motion to bring a cigarette, a drink of alcohol, a cup of coffee or a certain food to your lips, you are bringing something healthy to them instead.

**Noni Seed Oil Remedy #3**
1. Before you go to bed at night, tear a cotton ball in half.

2. Put a few drops of Noni seed oil on the cotton.

3. Lie down in bed and place the cotton on the point above the center of your upper lip, at the base of your nostrils.

4. Repeatedly press the cotton ball against this point. Breathe in the scent of Noni as you drift off to sleep.

This technique can be very relaxing and can be used to help you fall asleep at night if your cravings cause insomnia. Read more about the Scent of Noni on page 379.

**Use Noni Fruit Juice**
- Follow the Noni Protocol to Quit Smoking and for Addiction Relief on page 151.
- Try the Auto-dilution (page 133). In this case, spit out the Noni instead of swallowing it. Repeat the Auto-dilution as often as necessary.
- Use the Noni Headache Compress (page 297) as needed.
- Try the Noni Massage (page 309) or Noni for the Immune System (page 305).
- The Oral Detox (page 371) can help remove toxins from your mouth, head and brain. Be sure to spit out the Noni at the end of the Oral Detox procedure.
- Read the chapter on Using Intention with Noni (page 115). Use the techniques in this chapter and make a positive statement to affirm your freedom from addiction.

# MORE ABOUT NONI TECHNIQUES TO RELIEVE CRAVINGS AND WITHDRAWAL SYMPTOMS:

Practicing these techniques regularly will diminish your physical and psychological need for cigarettes or other addictive substances. However, it is critical that you also want to be free of your addiction. Then these techniques will offer more lasting results.

Try these techniques at least three times each, to find out which ones work best for you and which fit your lifestyle most conveniently.

Be sure to also follow the Noni Protocol to Quit Smoking and for Addiction Relief on page 151.

# -37-

# Noni Techniques
# for Alcohol Withdrawal

This technique supports a gradual withdrawal from alcohol. To quit "cold turkey," your body may need a great deal of additional support. You can receive this support by following the suggestions in the previous chapter, "Noni Techniques to Relieve Cravings and Withdrawal Symptoms."

## THE NONI TECHNIQUES FOR ALCOHOL WITHDRAWAL ARE FOR THOSE WHO:

- Are not yet ready to stop drinking, but would like to alleviate some of the negative effects of alcohol on their body.
- Would like to withdraw gradually.
- Would like to try an approach that allows them to continue drinking, but naturally reduces their craving for alcohol.

## HOW NONI CAN HELP YOU WITHDRAW FROM DRINKING ALCOHOL:

**Select from one of the following four techniques:**
- Make an agreement with yourself that before you have a glass of wine, bottle of beer, shot of whiskey or any other alcoholic drink, that you first drink one ounce of Noni fruit juice. This is the only rule: If you are going to drink

an alcoholic beverage, first drink one ounce of Noni. No matter what. Do this before each alcoholic beverage you have. If you go out to drink, take a flask of Noni with you.

Dehydration is a big problem for alcoholics and can cause innumerable symptoms, including an urge for more alcohol. So it is very important to drink water. The following three procedures are given as options.

- Follow the procedure in Enhancing Noni's Effects with Water (page 141).
- Follow the Noni Procedure for Serious Conditions #2 (page 87).
- Follow the procedure for Hydrating the Body with Noni (page 145).

## MORE ABOUT THE NONI TECHNIQUE FOR ALCOHOL WITHDRAWAL:

Taking an ounce of Noni before each alcoholic beverage may produce a number of different effects, or none at all. Your stomach may feel a little queasy, or you may get fully nauseated, which will naturally curb your drinking. You may get drunk more quickly, thereby decreasing your need for more alcohol. You may eventually get "turned off" by the alcohol and stop drinking. Over time, your desire for a drink should diminish. It may even go away after you take the ounce of Noni.

It is possible the alcoholic will find the taste of Noni so repulsive he or she may refuse to drink it. Adding an ounce of Noni to one or two ounces of an alcoholic beverage can make the taste tolerable. I know it sounds like an odd combination, but it really isn't so bad.

Noni's effect may be cumulative for some people. They may have to follow the above procedures for a while before they suddenly experience Noni's effects.

If you have a loved one who is an alcoholic, you may want to encourage him or her to follow the instructions in this chapter. However, alcoholics may feel threatened if you tell them the Noni will curb their desire for alcohol or help them stop drinking. Instead, tell them something else that is also completely true: tell them these procedures will help keep them healthy and alive. It will counteract some of the damage the alcohol is doing to their body. Assure them they don't have to quit drinking or drink any less. Then they may be more amenable to trying Noni. All an addict needs is to get enough Noni into their system, and their cells will begin to change. The cravings will eventually diminish in a natural, unstressful way.

Noni makes it easier to cut back the amount of alcohol that you drink, although quitting is most effective if you also summon your own desire and willpower.

After you have quit drinking, stabilize your body and ease withdrawal symptoms by using The Noni Techniques to Relieve Cravings and Withdrawal Symptoms (page 155) and following the Procedure for Serious Conditions #2 (page 87). As your body finds an addiction-free balance, gradually reduce the number of ounces of Noni you take each day. Remember to drink an ounce of Noni whenever the desire for alcohol arises and drink plenty of water, too.

# -38-

# Noni Technique for Food Addiction Relief

Addictions to foods such as coffee, chocolate or excessive sugar or carbohydrates are so commonplace that they have become a social norm. The degree of our addiction becomes apparent only when we try to make healthy changes to our diets.

## TRY THE NONI TECHNIQUE FOR FOOD ADDICTION RELIEF WHEN:

- You are allergic to a particular food, but do not have the willpower to avoid it.
- You are trying to lose weight by avoiding certain foods.
- You realize certain foods are harmful to your health, but are unable to remove them from your diet.

## HOW TO DO THE NONI TECHNIQUE FOR FOOD ADDICTION RELIEF:

1. Identify the food you would like to avoid. Select only one or two foods at a time.

2. Make an agreement with yourself that each time you reach for this food, you will first sip at least half a glass of a 1:8 Dilution of Noni. Here is how to make it:

   a. Pour one ounce of Noni fruit juice into a large drinking glass or one-quart jar.

    b.  Measure eight ounces of purified water in a measuring cup.

    c.  Swirl the glass so that the Noni is moving in a circular direction. Then pour the water into the Noni in a slow, steady, uninterrupted stream. Continue to swirl the glass for several seconds to mix the liquids together.

3.  Then you are free to eat the food or not.

Optional: If you still feel a desire for the food and sincerely want to avoid it, drink a second glass of the Dilution.

Make an agreement with yourself that you will follow this technique until you have gone at least fourteen days without eating the food(s) you chose in Step 1. After you drink enough of the 1:8 Dilution, your desire for this food should wane and the choice to avoid it will become an easier one to make.

## MORE ABOUT THE NONI TECHNIQUE FOR FOOD ADDICTION RELIEF:

The 1:8 Dilution is one of fourteen dilutions I have found that can be made from Noni fruit juice. Each dilution brings forth the restorative energies of Noni in a different way. The 1:8 Dilution has a particular affinity with the digestive system and the ability of the body to give and receive, or outflow and inflow. These metaphors are key to losing weight and detoxification, plus letting go of old and limiting concepts, mindsets and emotions, as well as receiving an inflow of health-giving energy and positive visions, affirmations, ideas and feelings.

The technique described in this chapter also works psychologically. It creates a span of time between a craving and the action of reaching for and eating the desired food. This time span is usually characterized by a sense of "unconsciousness" or complete lack of control. Preparing a Noni-water mixture and drinking it before eating the desired food lengthens this time span. Do what you can to lengthen it enough that you can gain control over the situation and choose another food—or an activity other than eating.

While you are drinking the Dilution, you may be battling the strong pull to eat the chosen food. Keep your commitment to yourself and to Noni. It may help to sip (page 39) the Dilution, drink it all at once (page 41), or hold each sip in your mouth for up to a minute before swallowing. It may also help to drink your Noni in a room other than the kitchen. Or go outside and drink it. Or drink it while telephoning a friend. Ideally, do something healthful, or emotionally or mentally rewarding in order to take your mind off the craved food. Be creative and experiment to see what works best for you.

The first few days of doing this technique, you may find yourself drinking many glasses of the 1:8 Dilution. Drink as many as you need and make sure your supply of Noni won't run out. Try not to be concerned that drinking this much liquid will increase your fluid retention. In most cases, the body retains fluid (as well as fat) as a result of dehydration. According to Dr. Batmanghelidj, "Water is the best natural diuretic that exists."[18]

If you do eat the chosen food after drinking the Dilution, you may find yourself eating less of it than you would otherwise. This is partly due to the fact that your stomach is full of Noni-water. The Noni will also supply your body with certain nutrients, the lack of which may be causing your body to crave certain foods. Noni's beneficial compounds also modify cell receptor sites. These sites will eventually attract more beneficial compounds, thereby reducing the body's physiological need for less healthful compounds. (To read about how Noni modifies receptor sites, see "Why Noni Works So Well for Addiction Relief" on page 154.)

---

[18] F. Batmanghelidj, M.D., *Water for Health, for Healing, for Life: You're not Sick, You're Thirsty,* (New York: Warner Books), p. 248.

When choosing a food in Step 1, be honest with yourself. If your problem is candy bars, for example, don't choose only one brand of candy bar to avoid...and then eat others. Choose all candy bars. If it is dairy products, include all dairy products, etc.

When following this technique, omit the regular daily servings of Noni that you might usually take. On those days you have no desire for the food chosen in Step 1, be sure to drink one or two servings of the 1:8 Dilution anyway.

The following techniques may also be helpful: A Noni Protocol to Quit Smoking and for Addiction Relief (page 151), Noni Techniques to Relieve Cravings and Withdrawal Symptoms (page 155), Enhancing Noni's Effects with Water (page 141), and the Noni Fasts (pages 171 and 175), the Auto-dilution (page 133) and the Oral Detox (page 371).

# -39-
# Using Noni as a Sleep Aid

Introducing the Bedtime Serving...

## NONI MAY HELP YOU FALL ASLEEP WHEN YOUR INSOMNIA IS RELATED TO:

- Anxiety.
- Emotional upset.
- High blood pressure.
- High blood sugar.
- Mental activity.
- Nervousness.
- Prescription medications.
- Stress.
- Too much caffeine in your bloodstream.

## HOW TO USE NONI AS A SLEEP AID:

1. When you are ready for bed, pour an ounce of Noni into a drinking glass.

2. Add an ounce of water. The amount does not have to be exact.

3. Take the Noni-water mixture into the bedroom. Get into bed and sip the Noni-water mixture slowly, perhaps while reading something that also relaxes you. You don't have to drink the entire amount.

# MORE ABOUT USING NONI AS A SLEEP AID:

I suggest adding one ounce of water because this amount is enough to prevent the stimulating effects of undiluted Noni, yet it is not enough to fill your bladder. You could also use the formula described in Chapter 66, "Noni to Enhance Dreams and Sleep" on page 261.

Drink the Noni-water mixture in the bedroom, so you can use Intention to correlate the serving with the sleep-inducing effect you would like to have (read more about Using Intention with Noni on page 115).

If you find that you consistently need less than the suggested serving, make smaller servings in the future. Noni commonly alleviates certain conditions that can cause insomnia. For example, if you have eaten carbohydrates or sugars late at night, the sugar in your bloodstream might keep you awake. Noni can lower blood sugar levels. If you can't sleep because of anxiety, stress or emotional upset, Noni can help calm your nervous system. If you are feeling jumpy and jittery from caffeine, Noni can neutralize some of the caffeine in your bloodstream. Some prescription medications also cause insomnia. Noni can help balance your body's chemistry, so you can sleep.

Noni fruit juice also boosts the performance of the pineal gland where a substance called melatonin is produced. Melatonin has a calming effect, induces sleep, allows you to dream, enhances deep REM sleep, which is when the body repairs itself and stimulates DNA in order to replace old cells with new ones.[19]

Try also The Noni Anti-stress Procedure (page 119), Using Noni to Enhance Dreams and Sleep (page 261) and Directing Noni with Breath and Focus (page 123). These techniques can also help you relax. Use only distilled water, spring water, purified tap water or untreated well water for this procedure. Chlorine, fluorine and other chemicals used to treat tap water can interfere with the body's ability to absorb and use Noni's beneficial compounds.

---

[19] Dr. Mona Harrison, *What Else Every Doctor Should Know: An Introduction to Noni and the Brains,* (Orem: Direct Source Publishing), 2002, p. 2, 35

# -40-
# The Noni Fast Method #1

During this fast, your entire diet will consist of Noni fruit juice.

## USE THE NONI FAST METHOD #1 IF YOU:

- Are relatively healthy and have the constitution to handle a fast.
- Enjoy fasting for general health maintenance.
- Would like the benefits of fasting, which include detoxification, improved mental clarity and greater health and well-being.
- Suspect your body may harbor parasites, yeast, viruses or infections and would like to use Noni to create an environment in your body unfavorable to them.
- Would like to correct poor eating habits.

## HOW TO FAST WITH NONI USING METHOD #1:

1. During this fast, replace all the food in your diet and all the liquid you would normally drink, with a special mixture of Noni and water called the 1:8 Dilution. To make one serving of this mixture:

    a. Pour one ounce of Noni fruit juice into a large drinking glass or one-quart jar.
    b. Measure eight ounces of purified water in a measuring cup.
    c. Swirl the glass so the Noni is moving in a circular direction. Then pour the water into the Noni in a

slow, steady, uninterrupted stream. Continue to swirl the glass for several seconds to mix the liquids together.

2. Drink eight to ten (or more) servings a day. If you feel hungry, sip a serving or two. Continue the fast for seven days.

3. On the eighth day, start breaking the fast by eating easily digestible foods. Such foods include fresh fruit and cooked vegetables. Continue to drink the 1:8 Dilution servings as before.

4. On the ninth day, drink six to eight servings of the 1:8 Dilution. Add a few more foods to your diet. Choose fruits, vegetables, whole grains and protein sources that work for you. Avoid junk food and overeating as your body is still recovering from the fast. Add two to four glasses of purified water to your diet.

5. On the tenth day, drink four to six servings of the 1:8 Dilution. Broaden your diet slightly more.

6. On the eleventh day, drink two to four servings of the 1:8 Dilution. Drink four to six glasses of purified water in addition to what you are now eating. Your diet should now be back to normal and hopefully you will have less desire for unhealthy foods.

7. On the twelfth day, the fast is over. Congratulations! Resume your Noni Maintenance Serving. Be sure to drink at least eight glasses of purified water each day.

# MORE ABOUT THE NONI FAST METHOD #1:

Instead of breaking the fast on the eighth day as suggested, you could continue the fast for another three days if you are feeling well and are enjoying the effects of the fast. On the other hand, a less intense version of the Noni Fast Method #1 would be to fast for three days instead of seven, and start breaking the fast on the fourth day.

Be sure to follow Steps 3 through 7, which guide you through ending the fast slowly. This is important if you want your body to let go of its cravings for certain foods, and therefore give you a chance to form new eating habits.

The Noni Fast is easier to do if you prepare several servings of the 1:8 Dilution ahead of time. As you finish making each serving, pour it into a pitcher. Store the pitcher in the refrigerator.

Fasting helps the body clean out toxins and rebalance all body systems. A Noni Fast does the same and more. Noni's special properties can enhance the immune system and help the body clear itself of yeast, fungus, parasites, bacteria and viruses. Noni also helps the body's enzymes, cell receptor sites and other protein molecules work more effectively and efficiently. Hence, a Noni Fast does more than clean out toxins; it also helps to repair and rebuild the body.

During this fast, you may experience cycles of both positive and negative cleansing reactions. The Noni Fast Method #1 can be intense. Consider doing the Noni Fast while you are on vacation from work, so you can get all the extra rest your body may need.

During the fast, consider using Noni Enemas (page 355) or a Noni Colonic Irrigation (page 358). These will help your body flush the toxins, parasites, and intestinal-wall buildup that the Noni Fast is helping your body to release. Parasites may be expelled into the toilet.

When you are doing a Noni Fast, omit the daily serving of Noni that you might usually take.

Before you start a fast of any kind, consult a health-care professional who can let you know if fasting is safe for someone in your health condition.

# -41-
# The Noni Fast Method #2

Here is another version of the Noni Fast.

## USE THE NONI FAST METHOD #2 IF YOU:

- Want the benefits of fasting, but don't want to stop eating.
- Want the benefits of fasting without having to change your lifestyle.
- Are not interested in initiating an uncomfortable cleansing reaction.
- Have health challenges that don't permit you to stop eating.

## HOW TO FAST WITH NONI USING METHOD #2:

1. During this fast, replace all the liquid in your diet— including water, coffee, tea, juice, soda pop, milk products, beer and other alcoholic beverages—with a special mixture of Noni and water. To make one serving of this special mixture, which is also called a 1:12 Dilution:

   a. Pour an ounce of Noni fruit juice into a quart-size jar.
   b. Use a two-cup measuring cup to measure twelve ounces (one-and-a-half cups) of purified water.
   c. Swirl the jar so the Noni is moving in a circular direction. Then pour the water into the Noni in a slow, steady, uninterrupted stream. Continue to swirl the glass for several seconds to mix the liquids together.

One serving of this mixture consists of thirteen ounces of liquid (one ounce of Noni plus twelve ounces of water).

2.  Drink six or more servings of this mixture each day. (Six servings is a little over nine-and-a-half cups of liquid.) Start with one before breakfast. Spread the others throughout the day, but drink one whenever you are thirsty.

3.  You may continue to eat during this fast. Focus your diet on fresh vegetables and fruits, whole grains and protein foods that work for you. Avoid refined sugar, white flour, saturated fat, chocolate, preservatives, food additives and processed foods.

## MORE ABOUT THE NONI FAST METHOD #2:

Try this fast for three days at a time. Fasting any longer may initiate a cleansing reaction. If a cleansing reaction does occur, drink more of the 1:12 Dilution to help your body flush the toxins that have been released.

While doing this fast, give yourself more rest and try deep breathing exercises. Do the Noni Anti-Stress Procedure (page 119). Try the Noni Enema (page 355).

The Noni Fast #2 is easier to do if you prepare several servings of the 1:12 Dilution ahead of time. As you finish making each one, pour it into a pitcher and store the pitcher in the refrigerator.

People often lose weight while fasting. Since foods are not limited with this fast, however, weight loss may or may not occur. If you would like to lose weight, try sipping an entire serving of the 1:12 Dilution when you feel hungry. This may reduce your appetite.

When you are doing a Noni Fast, omit the daily serving of Noni you might otherwise be taking.

# –42–
# A Noni
# Detoxification Program

This cleansing program naturally urges the body to release toxins with the nutritional support that only Noni can provide.

## USE THE NONI
## DETOXIFICATION PROGRAM IF YOU:

- Are relatively healthy.
- Would like the benefits of fasting without having to cut out food from your diet.
- Would like to carefully control the detoxification process.

## HOW TO INITIATE
## A DETOXIFICATION WITH NONI:

To do this program, you take a sip of Noni at regular intervals for a chosen number of hours each day, for a chosen number of days. For example, you might sip Noni every thirty minutes between noon and 5:00 PM for three days.

1. Read about the Three Variables of the Noni Detoxification Program below. Then choose the variable you want to use: 1) the time interval between Noni sips, 2) the number of hours per day you want to do the program, and 3) for how many days you would like to do the program. During the program, you can modify these selections to control your

detoxification process as describe in the section "More about the Noni Detoxification Program." Use the spaces below to write down your initial choices.

What time interval between sips? _____

How many hours per day? _____

How many days? _____

2.  When you are ready to begin the program, pour some Noni into a drinking glass. Estimate how much you might need for the day. You may have to add more later, or if you have poured too much, put the glass in the refrigerator and save it for the next day.

3.  Take your first sip and mark what time it is.

4.  Set a clock timer such as an alarm clock or oven timer to alert you when to take your next serving based on the time interval you chose in Step 1.

5.  When the timer rings, take your next sip.

6.  Repeat Steps 4 and 5 for as many hours as you have chosen in Step 1.

## THE THREE VARIABLES OF THE NONI DETOXIFICATION PROGRAM:

**The Time Interval:**
This can be as frequent as a few minutes or as long as one hour. The more frequent the intervals, the more intense the detoxification will be and the more attention you will have to give to the procedure.

**How Many Hours per Day you want to do the Program:**
This can be as short as about thirty minutes or as long as about twelve hours. However, it must be long enough that you are able to drink at least five servings. Select a duration that you can commit to each day for the number of days that you want to do this program. While doing the program, if you begin to feel that the detoxification is becoming too intense, cut back the amount of time in which you are sipping Noni that day.

**How Many Days:**
The number of days you would like to continue this program can be one day or up to about fourteen. You may choose to modify this number during the program depending on how you feel.

## MORE ABOUT THE NONI DETOXIFICATION PROGRAM:

The Noni Detoxification Program is powerful because taking a healthful substance like Noni at predefined intervals establishes a rhythm that can reset the body's own rhythms. A healthy body is accustomed to regularity of all its functions and cycles. As we age or as our health declines, our rhythms and cycles break down. They weaken and become less reliable. Cellular processes become less organized and less efficient.

The Noni Detoxification Program forces the body into rhythm by regularly presenting it with Noni. The body responds very quickly to this rhythm. It uses the rhythm like a template that encourages the body's natural rhythms to tighten up and become more regular. Regular rhythm encourages the cellular processes to become more organized and efficient.

Do not underestimate the power of this program. It can bring on an intense cleansing reaction as your body adjusts to a renewed rhythm and a higher level of health. It doesn't take long before your body begins to detoxify. For example, your bowels may become more active, your appetite may decrease, and you may become either more restful or more energized depending on what is going on in your body at the time. (See a list of possible cleansing reactions on pages 410 and 415.)

Fortunately, you can control how intensely this cleansing occurs. To intensify a detoxification, simply increase the amount of time per day that you do the program.

To alleviate cleansing reactions, stop the program and take no more Noni that day. The next day, increase the time interval between Noni sips. Stay faithful to this new schedule for at least one day. You may need to continue adjusting the interval until you find one that allows your body to tighten its rhythms without your having to suffer uncomfortable cleansing reactions. Remember, if you modify the time interval, do so only in the morning and follow that same interval throughout the day.

Avoid changing the interval more than two or three times. You need to trust your initial choice, though the procedure does give you room to modify that choice. I believe your body's needs will speak through your intuition and mental decision-making process as you choose which interval to use.

# -43-
# A Gentle Noni
# Detoxification Program

This gentle detoxification program is designed for those who are extremely sensitive to herbs and supplements (such as Noni) that can benefit the body, but that also have a cleansing effect.

## TRY THE GENTLE NONI DETOXIFICATION PROGRAM FOR:

- Chemical toxicity.
- Electromagnetic energy sensitivity.
- Systemic yeast.
- Heavy metal poisoning.
- Parasites.

## HOW TO DO THE GENTLE NONI DETOXIFICATION PROGRAM:

1. Prepare a Noni-water mixture called the 1:12 Dilution. To make this mixture:

   a. Pour an ounce of Noni into a one-quart mason jar.
   b. Measure twelve ounces (one and a half cups of water) in a two cup measuring cup.
   c. Swirl the jar so the Noni is moving in a circular direction. Meanwhile, pour the water into the Noni in a steady, uninterrupted stream. Continue to swirl the jar for another few seconds to mix the liquids together.

2.   Do each of the following every day:
     •   Take a small sip of 1:12 Dilution to use the Auto-dilution (page 133). Do the Auto-dilution once a day and over time increase to three or four times a day.
     •   Do a body splash as follows. Pour about one-half cup of the 1:12 Dilution and bring it with you into the bathroom. Before you take a shower, remove your clothes, stand in the shower stall and splash the 1:12 Dilution all over your body. Massage it gently into your skin until it dries. Taking a shower will terminate the effects of this procedure, giving your immune system a boost that lasts just as long as the 1:12 Dilution is on your skin. If you want the effects to linger, do this technique after you have showered and towel-dried.
     •   Also try a Noni Enema (page 355) using just the one recipe of 1:12 Dilution. It will be a small enema as far as liquid volume is concerned, but the impact of most importance is the energetic effect of the 1:12 Dilution. Introducing the dilution into your bowels should help the entire body put more focus on elimination through the intestinal tract.

3.   As you become more comfortable with the 1:12 Dilution and are able to stay in balance with the Auto-dilution, body splash and enema, try drinking one teaspoonful of the 1:12 Dilution. Try one serving a day and over time increase to about three servings a day. Keep your servings small. Large servings may upset your state of balance and are unnecessary for your condition. Eventually, as your body gets stronger, you will be able to drink more Noni and handle a proportionately greater detoxification in balance.

# MORE ABOUT THE GENTLE NONI DETOXIFICATION PROGRAM:

This program is based on a mixture of Noni and water called the 1:12 Dilution. This Dilution brings forth the particular Noni restorative energy that integrates and helps to orchestrate the entire body as a whole. This includes the body's physical and nonphysical parts, processes and energy flows.

Of all the Noni dilutions, I believe the 1:12 Dilution is best suited for gradual detoxification because it alerts all the cells in the body to Noni's presence. The cells are then able to work together in greater harmony and efficiency to respond to the opportunity for greater health that is being presented.

Meanwhile, Noni beneficial compounds support the body while it cleanses. These compounds strengthen the cells, improve the immune system and bring new vitality to the cells, giving them the strength to let go toxins in a balanced way.

The point is to detoxify the body gradually and avoid uncomfortable cleansing reactions. Life is for living. Noni has shown me it is possible to live in a healthier state while the body naturally fulfills its processes of elimination like a computer program running in the background—essential, but not in the forefront of attention.

# -44-
## Noni Tea

Adding hot water to Noni will not hurt the beneficial compounds in the juice. On the contrary, I believe the body absorbs Noni's beneficial compounds more readily when the Noni is taken at room temperature or warmer.

### DRINK NONI TEA:

- At the onset of flu-like symptoms.
- As a tonic before or during flu season.
- As a tonic before or during times of unusual stress.
- For immune deficiency conditions, in place of regular servings of Noni.
- For throat conditions including sore throat, swollen glands and tonsillitis.
- To help relieve the symptoms of colds and flu.
- To help you relax after a stressful day.
- Just for fun.

### HOW TO MAKE NONI TEA:

1. Pour one ounce of Noni fruit juice into a mug. (Don't use plastic or paper cups.)

2. Boil about a cup of purified water. (Use a glass, enamel or stainless steel pot.)

3. Pour exactly five ounces of the hot water into a glass measuring cup. Hold the cup at eye-level to make sure

the measurement is accurate.

4.  Swirl the mug so the Noni is moving in a circular motion. Meanwhile, pour the five ounces of hot water into the mug in a slow, steady, uninterrupted stream. Continue swirling the mug for a few seconds more to mix the liquids together.

5.  Sip, as you would drink tea.

## MORE ABOUT NONI TEA:

One serving of Noni Tea consists of five ounces of hot water added to one ounce of Noni fruit juice. This is called a 1:5 Dilution. The 1:5 Dilution activates the Noni restorative energy that protects the body and strengthens its defense mechanisms.

To double the serving, add ten ounces of hot water to two ounces of Noni fruit juice. You will need an extra-large mug for this. Double servings of Noni Tea are especially helpful at the onset of flu-like symptoms and may also be used for the Procedure for Acute Conditions, on page 75.

To make Noni Tea use spring water, distilled water, filtered water or pure well water. Do not use chlorinated or fluoridated water. These chemicals may interfere with the body's ability to absorb Noni's beneficial compounds.

Hot Noni Tea feels wonderfully soothing on a sore throat. If your Noni Tea cools off, it is still beneficial to drink. Check the temperature of Noni Tea before giving it to children to make sure it isn't too hot for them.

For colds and flu, drink Noni Tea three to five times a day. See also Noni Ear Drops (page 349) and Noni Nose Drops (page 367). For bronchial conditions and coughing, try a Noni Poultice (page 229) on the chest, over the lungs.

# -45-
# The Noni Tonic

The Noni Tonic boosts the immune system and helps the body handle stressful situations.

## TAKE A NONI TONIC BEFORE POTENTIALLY STRESSFUL SITUATIONS SUCH AS:

- Birthdays, holidays, or anytime you plan to eat greater quantities of food, or more sugar, fat and refined foods than usual.
- Domestic upheavals, from family squabbles to divorce.
- Events that may be particularly stressful, such as exams, presentations, speeches and competitions.
- Recitals and other on-stage performances.
- Surgery.
- The beginning of school (or day care for young children).
- Traveling, especially out of the country.
- Visits to the doctor's, dentist's or attorney's office.

## HOW TO TAKE A NONI TONIC:

A Noni Tonic consists of drinking a serving of Noni Tea three or four times a day, preferably on an empty stomach. To make Noni Tea, see page 185.

1. Take the Noni Tonic before the anticipated event:
   - Start a few days before one-day events.
   - Start two weeks before particularly stressful events, such as surgery.

2. Take a serving of Noni Tea immediately before the event begins and another as soon as possible afterwards.

3. After the event, continue taking the Noni Tonic until things calm down. Then return to your usual Noni serving size.

Continue to take the Noni Tonic during extended stressful situations, such as the breaking up of a marriage or especially rough times at work.

## MORE ABOUT THE NONI TONIC:

When people are under stress, their immune system suffers and Noni Tea can help. Noni Tea is preferable over undiluted Noni fruit juice because it boosts the immune system from two approaches. First, Noni beneficial compounds naturally boost the immune system (you receive this benefit just by drinking Noni fruit juice). Second, the 1:5 Dilution of Noni Tea activates the Noni restorative energy that can protect the body and strengthen its defense mechanisms.

Teenagers can take the same amounts as adults. Give older children half a serving of Noni Tea on the same schedule as suggested above. Give young children sips of Noni Tea several times a day. If your children refuse to drink Noni Tea, try giving it to them cold. Do not add ice as that will disrupt the Noni-water ratio. See page 198 for a list of creative ways to give Noni to children. When preparing for surgery, remember to also take the Noni Trauma Serving (page 95). If you are seriously ill and usually drink more than three or four ounces of Noni a day, substitute each ounce of Noni you usually take with one serving of Noni Tea.

# -46-

# Noni in Foods

To obtain the full benefit from Noni's beneficial compounds, it is best to drink Noni on an empty stomach. But sometimes this can be too much to ask of children or other family members who may object to Noni's taste—or even to the idea of taking supplements. An option is to include Noni in Foods. Though the stomach's digestive juices may destroy some of Noni's beneficial compounds, other compounds still work, as Noni is a proven digestive aid and Antacid Substitute (page 195) when taken after meals.

## INCLUDE NONI IN FOODS WHEN:

- Adding Noni fruit juice to foods may be the only way a child will take Noni orally.
- You feel nauseated when you try to drink Noni.
- You want the benefits of Noni, but don't care for the taste.
- You have a sensitive stomach or a toxicity condition.
- You want to add Noni to your family's meals as a tasty and healthful ingredient.

# SOME IDEAS FOR ADDING NONI FRUIT JUICE TO FOODS:

## Sauces and Spreads:
- Mix one-half to one ounce of Noni fruit juice with one-quarter to one-half cup of blueberry sauce. Pour this on cheesecake, pancakes or waffles.
- Beat together two to three ounces of Noni fruit juice with a half cup of softened butter. The butter will turn lavender-pink. Store in the refrigerator. Spread on breads and muffins.
- Add one tablespoonful of Noni fruit juice to the jelly jar and mix. Try this for making peanut butter and jelly sandwiches.
- Mix one ounce of Noni fruit juice with one ounce of tahini or peanut butter. Mix in two to four teaspoonfuls of soy sauce to taste. Use as a sauce over vegetables and grains.
- Combine equal parts of Noni fruit juice, peanut butter and maple syrup to cover almost anything.
- Beat eight ounces of softened cream cheese with one ounce of Noni for a lightly colored lavender spread. Add two ounces for a slightly darker color and a softer spread. Use on crackers and sprinkle with dried dill weed.

## Soups:
- Add one, two or three teaspoonfuls of Noni fruit juice per serving of canned or homemade soup after cooking.

## Salads and Dressings:
- Add an ounce or two of Noni to any commercial salad dressing bottle. Shake well before serving. Noni is particularly tasty in vinaigrettes.

- Add a teaspoonful or more of Noni per serving of fruit salad.
- Mix shredded carrots with raisins, coconut, honey, cinnamon and Noni fruit juice. Add one or two tablespoonfuls of Noni per cup of shredded carrots.
- Try "Tahitian Tuna Salad" using tuna, mayonnaise, chopped carrots and celery, coconut, pineapple and Noni fruit juice. Add one tablespoonful of Noni per cup of tuna salad.
- Make "Noni Compoti" with canned pear halves that are filled with a teaspoonful of Noni fruit juice then a dollop of cottage cheese. Top with a maraschino cherry.

## Grains:

- After cooking white rice, add an ounce or two of Noni fruit juice. Use a fork to fluff the rice and mix in the juice. The Noni will give the rice a light purple color.
- Noni fruit juice may also be added to cooked whole grains. Add sesame seeds and raisins to emphasize the fruity flavor.
- Make "Rigatoni Noni" using cooked rigatoni noodles. Add Noni fruit juice to heated tomato sauce. Mix with the noodles. Top with grated Parmesan cheese. Adding Noni to tomato sauce is a foolproof way to hide Noni's flavor. Try adding a tablespoonful or more per serving, and your family may never know it's there.

## Vegetables:

- Mash sweet potatoes, and then add butter, honey, cinnamon and a teaspoonful or two of Noni fruit juice per serving.

- Add Noni fruit juice to cooked carrots, green beans and onions after they've been cooked. Use a teaspoonful or two of Noni per serving.
- Sauté leafy greens and mushrooms. When done cooking, add a teaspoonful of Noni fruit juice per serving.

**Meat/Fish/Poultry/Tofu/Tempeh Marinades and Sauces:**
Cooking foods that have been marinated in Noni may destroy some of Noni's beneficial compounds. So use Noni in marinades for flavor, and for its tenderizing effect on meats and poultry.

- Try a marinade made with one ounce of Noni fruit juice, two ounces of orange juice concentrate, two teaspoonfuls of soy sauce (or more to taste), one ounce of berry juice (raspberry, cherry or blueberry), and two ounces of finely chopped red onion. Garnish the cooked dish with fresh berries in season.
- Try one or two tablespoonfuls of Noni in your favorite marinade recipe.
- Dip cooked shrimp in a mixture of one ounce of horseradish, one ounce of ketchup, and a tablespoonful of Noni fruit juice. The Noni significantly reduces the sharpness of the horseradish.
- Try a sauce made from two or three cloves of crushed garlic, one ounce of Noni fruit juice and one ounce of soy sauce.
- Add a tablespoonful of Noni fruit juice per quarter-cup to half-cup of barbecue sauce.
- Sprinkle one tablespoonful of Noni fruit juice over each cup of stuffing, after it has been cooked and removed from the turkey.

**Desserts:**

- Mix equal parts of Noni fruit juice and chocolate or strawberry sauce for an ice cream topping.
- Make homemade ice cream flavored with Noni fruit juice and other fruits and berries. Or simply use Noni with other fruits and berries as a topping for store-bought ice cream or frozen yogurt. Noni fruit juice tastes quite good over vanilla or chocolate ice cream.
- Add fruit chunks, honey, and a teaspoonful or two of Noni fruit juice to plain, unsweetened yogurt. Sprinkle with nuts or wheat germ.
- Add one tablespoonful of Noni to spiced apple cider.
- Sprinkle one to three ounces of Noni fruit juice on top of fruit pies, cobblers and bread pudding after cooking.
- Make buttercream frosting using butter and confectioner's sugar. Use Noni instead of milk or cream. The Noni will color the frosting a pretty lavender-pink.
- Make a fruity Noni gelatin dessert by dissolving one package of unflavored gelatin in two cups of a natural fruit juice. Heat while stirring until the gelatin is dissolved. Pour the hot liquid into serving bowls. Add chopped bananas, grapes, apples or other favorite fruit. Then add one teaspoonful of Noni fruit juice per serving. Put the gelatin in the refrigerator to set. If you pour Noni into a light-colored fruit juice and stir, the fruit juice will become a darker color throughout. If you pour the Noni in very gently and don't stir, the Noni pulp will form a pretty "cloud" which settles at the bottom of the bowl.

## MORE ABOUT NONI IN FOODS:

The therapeutic effects of Noni added to foods will be less immediate and not as strong as Noni fruit juice taken by itself on an empty stomach. The amounts of Noni given in the recipes in this chapter are suggestions only. Adjust the amount to suit your taste and preference.

How much Noni you can add to a recipe depends on how well the juice combines with the other ingredients and how important it is to mask Noni's flavor. Generally, recipes can incorporate a teaspoonful to a tablespoonful of Noni per serving.

It is best to add Noni to foods after they have been cooked. Although Noni fruit juice has been pasteurized during processing, the heating temperature used is carefully regulated so Noni's beneficial compounds remain intact. However, cooking can easily raise the temperature beyond the acceptable limits and destroy these compounds.

Noni affects various foods in different ways. For example, Noni fruit juice lends an attractive light purple color to some white and light colored foods, such as white rice and potatoes. It can give other foods a brownish tinge, which may not be appetizing. Noni enhances the flavor of some foods, such as garlic, and subdues the flavor of others, such as horseradish. Some foods, like tomato sauce, mask Noni's flavor.

If you aren't accustomed to eating sugar, then Noni might help you handle its effects. Either add the Noni to the dessert recipe, or drink it after eating the sugary food. Of course, this does not give license to diabetics or other sugar-sensitive people to eat foods they should otherwise avoid. But this tip can be helpful at birthdays and other holiday occasions.

When you are making a large recipe with many servings, you may want to know how much Noni you need. Multiply the amount of Noni you would like each person to receive by the number of servings in your recipe. This will give you the total amount of Noni to add.

# -47-
# The Noni Antacid Substitute

Although Noni does not work in the same way as regular antacids, the results are often just as relieving.

## TRY THE NONI
## ANTACID SUBSTITUTE FOR:

- Heartburn.
- Indigestion.
- Stomach distress from overeating.
- In addition, if you are relatively healthy but unaccustomed to certain foods like refined sugar, meat or "junk" food, Noni may help your body handle these foods on those special occasions when you do eat them.

## HOW TO USE NONI
## AS AN ANTACID SUBSTITUTE:

1. Drink one tablespoonful of Noni following your meal, before or after symptoms arise.

2. If you don't feel better after a few minutes, try drinking another tablespoonful.

# MORE ABOUT THE
# NONI ANTACID SUBSTITUTE:

The effects of taking Noni before a meal verses after it, are different. Noni taken before a meal, on an empty stomach, will help the underlying cause of stomach distress. Taking the Noni Antacid Substitute after a meal will better address the symptoms of a stomach condition.

For chronic indigestion, try the Procedure for Chronic Conditions (page 79), which suggests taking three ounces of Noni a day. Take one of these three ounces a few minutes before each meal. Then eat mindfully. If you still feel distress afterwards, take a tablespoonful or more of Noni after the meal. Eventually, you may not need the Noni Antacid Substitute any more.

Taking an ounce of Noni before each meal can help curb your appetite if you tend to overeat, especially if you drink it with a glass of water.

The Noni Fast Method #2 (page 175) is another approach to dealing with chronic indigestion and heartburn. See also Hydrating with Noni (page 145).

# —48—

## Giving Noni to Children

"You want me to drink, what?"

## BABIES AND YOUNG CHILDREN:

Healthy babies, toddlers and children up to the age of about eight or nine probably don't need to drink Noni fruit juice every day. They might even resist the juice when you try to give it to them. If they are healthy, trust their body's innate intelligence. Offer them Noni when you drink yours to accustom them to a routine and lifestyle that includes Noni fruit juice. If they refuse to drink any, at least let them see that you drink Noni daily.

At times, you may want to insist your children take Noni. For example when they get sick or as a tonic to support their immune system before a vacation, before the holidays, before school begins or after they have eaten something very sweet. Some creative ways to make Noni more appealing to children are listed below.

Youngsters who become ill or injured will have a specific need for Noni, and tend to take it readily and eagerly. In this case, give them as much Noni fruit juice as they will drink— within reason. Use topical applications freely. One serving may be all they need to alleviate relatively mild conditions.

Seriously ill children can follow the Procedures for Serious Conditions (page 83 and 87) or for Life-Threatening Conditions (page 91). Give babies and toddlers one-quarter of each serving suggested for adults. Older children can take one-half of each serving. But give more if they are willing and eager to drink it.

Drinking Noni fruit juice may soften a child's stools. But

this can be helpful if a child is taking antibiotics, which often cause constipation. You will have to weigh the temporary inconvenience of loose stools with the tremendous benefits the child will receive from taking Noni.

## TWO SECRETS FOR SUCCESSFULLY GIVING NONI TO CHILDREN:

1. Make it fun.
2. Don't make a fuss over it.

## CREATIVE WAYS TO GIVE NONI TO BABIES AND CHILDREN

- Mix Noni with another fruit juice.
- Make homemade frozen juice-pops with Noni fruit juice mixed with other fruit juices.
- Mix Noni with applesauce, cottage cheese or other favorite foods.
- Give Noni to infants with an eyedropper or add it to their bottles.
- Try giving Noni to children while they take a bath. This can be fun, and if any Noni is spilled, their clothes won't get stained.
- Let children drink their Noni with a straw.
- Give little children their Noni in a colorful container that is usually not used for drinking, such as a toy stacking cup.
- Let them choose a special cup from your cupboard, or buy a special one that will be used only for drinking Noni.
- Play a pretend game with your youngster. Build a bird's nest with sheets and towels. Pretend your child is a baby

bird and you are the father or mother bird. What do baby birds eat? Worms, of course! Pretend you are giving your baby bird a worm, using an eyedropper filled with Noni fruit juice. Worms taste yucky, but baby birds love them. Show your child how baby birds tilt their heads back and open their mouths for their parents to put in food. After a baby bird eats a worm, she ruffles her little wings and opens her mouth for more (ruffling her "wings" may distract your child from the Noni's taste).

- Let them drink straight from the Noni bottle. Though you won't know exactly how much they drink, their body's intelligence will likely inspire them to take as much as they need.
- It helps if your children know they are welcome to drink Noni whenever they want to. I often find my seven-year old, Kellan, "sneaking" Noni after eating too much or having too many sweets. She knows the Noni helps her tummy feel better. Of course, I don't say anything and pretend not to notice.
- If your child is old enough, explain how Noni can help them. Noni fruit juice can help their bodies fight germs. It can help them be strong and healthy, so they can feel better again sooner.
- Get on your hands and knees and beg. (Just kidding!)
- If a child flat-out refuses to drink Noni fruit juice, you might apply a Noni Tummy Treatment instead. If necessary, this may be done at night while the child is sleeping. It can also be applied each time a baby is diapered.
- Let drinking Noni fruit juice become a natural part of your family's daily routine. Use Noni topical and internal applications often. Let Noni be one of the first things that comes to mind when you think about using a home remedy.

When I asked my eight-year old daughter, Aria Ray, if I could apply Noni Paste to a wound, she was concerned that it might hurt. Then she thought about it and said, "How could Noni hurt? It's just a juice!"

## PRE-TEENS AND TEENAGERS:

When children enter the pre-teen and teen years, they could benefit from a daily serving of Noni fruit juice. It may ease the many transitions their bodies are making.

If teens aren't forced to drink Noni, they will be more willing to take it. Still, they may watch what Noni does for their parents first before they try it themselves. Let them know the juice is available for them.

Tell them Noni can be used both orally and topically to help some conditions that are of particular concern to teens. For example, Noni can help clear the skin, stabilize mood swings, ease growing pains, enhance athletic performance and speed recovery time for athletic injuries.

Teenagers may follow the same procedures and take the same servings as adults. Teens who weigh less than one hundred pounds can take half the suggested amounts.

# -49-

# The Sick Day
# Prevention Serving

This serving is for the whole family. Take it in addition to your regular daily servings of Noni.

## TRY THE NONI SICK DAY
## PREVENTION SERVING WHEN:

- Someone in your family has been exposed to a contagious illness.
- Someone in your family shows the first signs or symptoms of the flu or other acute illness.
- Your children seem more tired and cranky than usual. (This can be a sign of a weakened or stressed immune system, which is a precursor to illness.)
- You sense that someone in your family may be "coming down with something." You may not have any physical evidence to support this suspicion, but parents should trust their intuition. It can only help to drink extra Noni, just in case.

## HOW TO USE NONI TO PREVENT SICK DAYS:

1. Immediately give a Sick-Day Prevention Serving to the family member who is showing signs of illness. Also give one to everyone else in the family. Ideally, this serving should be consumed all at once (page 41).

2. Later that day, family members should take a second Sick-Day Prevention Serving.

3. Continue to have everyone in the family take two or three Sick-Day Prevention Servings per day for a few days, or until everyone in the family is feeling better.

## HOW MUCH IS A SICK DAY PREVENTION SERVING?

- For adults and teenagers, two ounces.
- For preteens, one or two ounces.
- For children, one ounce.
- And for babies and toddlers, one-half ounce (or one tablespoonful).

## MORE ABOUT USING NONI TO PREVENT SICK DAYS:

The immune support and antibacterial, antiviral and antifungal properties that Noni can provide should boost the immune system of everyone in the family to clear up infection before it spreads throughout the family. It should also reduce the potential severity of the sickness.

Sometimes children who are ill or fighting illness intuitively know Noni can help them and will ask for more. Feel free to give them as much as they want, within reasonable limits (perhaps about one-half cup per serving). When the illness has passed, however, they should return to their usual Maintenance Serving (page 63).

The Sick-Day Prevention Serving should be taken in addition to your regularly daily serving of Noni.

# -50-
# The Family Serving

This is a simple way to add Noni fruit juice to your family's diet.

## TRY THIS TECHNIQUE
## WHEN YOU OR YOUR FAMILY:

- Often forget to take a daily serving of Noni.
- Object to Noni's taste.
- Are accustomed to drinking water or iced tea from a pitcher, or juice from a container kept in the refrigerator.

## TRY THE FAMILY SERVING WHEN:

- You are using Noni for health maintenance.
- It doesn't matter exactly how much Noni each of your family members is getting. (When someone gets sick, please see The Sick Day Prevention Serving on page 201.)
- Your family typically pours from the same pitcher or container of water, iced tea or juice.

## HOW TO PROVIDE THE FAMILY SERVING:

1. Decide how much Noni to add to a pitcher or container of beverage. A guideline is to add from one tablespoonful to three ounces of Noni per two-quart pitcher. Start with the smaller amount and each week increase the serving.

2.  Decide if and how you will tell your family members about the "hidden" Noni. If you think your children will be reluctant to drink anything with "something strange" (like Noni) added to it, you may prefer not to tell them and see if they notice it themselves first. Noni fruit juice is easily disguised in iced tea and other fruit juices.

## MORE ABOUT PROVIDING YOUR FAMILY WITH THE FAMILY SERVING:

How much Noni you add to the pitcher may depend on
*   The size of the pitcher.
*   How open your family is to taking their servings of Noni inside another beverage.
*   How important it is to "hide" the presence of Noni in the beverage.
*   How much of this other beverage your family usually drinks each day, and approximately how much Noni you would like your family to consume.

If you do not typically prepare a beverage to be available in a community pitcher, try it and see how your family likes the idea. They may appreciate the convenience.

# -51-
## Keeping Noni
## a Family Friend

Here are some ways to keep Noni a family friend, even after the initial excitement of using Noni wears off.

## THE IDEAS IN THIS CHAPTER CAN BE HELPFUL FOR:

- All members of the family.
- General health maintenance.
- The long-time Noni enthusiast.

## HOW TO KEEP NONI A FAMILY FRIEND:

Here are some ideas for incorporating Noni into a family lifestyle:

- Make a ritual of giving everyone in the family their daily serving of Noni at the same time and place.
- When injuries occur, remember Noni. Refer to the chapter on Noni First Aid (page 281).
- Let your children observe how you reach for Noni after minor cuts and burns, and other needs.
- Become familiar with the topical and internal Noni procedures described in this book. Experiment with them and find out which ones work best for you. When

a situation arises that may be helped by one of these procedures, you will be more comfortable using it if you have already experimented with it beforehand.

- Let your children help you make and apply various topical applications including Noni Paste, Noni Poultices and Noni Compresses.
- Make it a habit to turn to Noni whenever a health condition arises.
- At the first sign of colds or flu, make it a habit to take extra servings of Noni or make Noni Tea (page 185).
- Use the Family Serving technique (page 203).
- Keep at least two extra bottles of Noni available for emergencies, when extra servings may be required.
- *Think* Noni. Make this your motto, so whenever a health condition arises, you will naturally remember to think about how you can use Noni.
- When Noni doesn't seem to be working as before, keep the faith, be creative, and try a new way to use Noni. See the chapter on "Ways to Enhance the Effects of Noni" on page 397.
- Keep this book handy for reference.

## MORE ABOUT KEEPING NONI A FAMILY FRIEND:

Noni is here to help you and your family. It is Nature's Gift. All you have to do is be willing to try it, use it, and keep looking for new ways it can help you. It is important to be creative and flexible with Noni and be ever willing to experiment and try new ways to work with it. The ideas in this book can get you started.

# -52-
# Giving Noni to Cats and Dogs

The following tips for giving Noni fruit juice to cats and dogs are not meant to replace your veterinarian's care. Use them in addition to the therapies your vet suggests.

Our pets can benefit from the beneficial compounds in Noni just as much as human beings can. Generally, the effects of Noni on their bodies will be the same as the effects on ours. Because their body size is much smaller, serving size amounts need to be adjusted accordingly.

Young, healthy cats and dogs probably don't need a Maintenance Serving, but if you get them accustomed to Noni as kittens and puppies, they will be more agreeable to taking Noni if ever their health requires it.

Definitely consider giving older pets a Maintenance Serving. Animals often hide their aches and pains, or if they do try to communicate how they feel, we can miss what they're trying to tell us. A Noni Maintenance Serving can alleviate mild symptoms, boost their immune system and help prevent disease.

## TIPS FOR GIVING NONI TO CATS:

A Maintenance Serving for cats can be about one-half to one teaspoonful of Noni per day. Add this amount to your cat's food. If necessary, start with one-eighth teaspoonful and gradually increase the serving as your cat becomes accustomed to it. If you usually give your cat dry food, try a serving of Noni in wet food and she will love it.

When measuring servings of one teaspoonful or less, start by pouring some Noni into a medicine cup. Then pour the Noni from the medicine cup into the measuring spoon. This way the Noni is less likely to spill. One idea is to pour one ounce of your own daily serving and share a teaspoonful of it with your cat.

If your cat becomes ill, but is still eating, increase the daily serving size of Noni that you put in her food. If she is unable to eat, refuses the higher serving size in her food, or needs to take Noni on an empty stomach to receive the full effect of Noni's beneficial compounds, you will have to inject the serving into the back of her mouth. To do this you will need an eyedropper or small plastic syringe tube. Plastic syringe tubes can be found in pet stores. They are typically used to hand feed small animals and baby parrots.

Syringe tubes have markings to identify serving amounts. On the other hand, eyedroppers come in different sizes and may be unmarked. If using an eyedropper, pre-measure the total daily amount of Noni you want to give her. Use the eyedropper to draw from this amount throughout the day. Your cat may prefer Noni at room temperature, so keep the serving on the countertop. A day outside the refrigerator won't spoil it.

Giving Noni to cats via an eyedropper or syringe can be challenging and will take practice. Tip your cat's head up and gently pry open her teeth before injecting the Noni into the back of her throat. To help her swallow the Noni, stimulate her swallowing reflex by stroking her throat downward with the side of your finger.

Some cats won't mind having Noni injected into their mouth. Others won't stand for it. If your cat is still strong enough to bathe herself, here is another way to give her Noni.

1. Fill a clean eyedropper or plastic syringe with a serving of Noni fruit juice.

**Optional:** Hold the syringe in a bowl or sink full of hot water to warm the juice. Most cats probably don't care whether or not you warm their Noni. Those who are very ill might appreciate it.

2. While petting your cat with one hand, hold the syringe with the other hand. Slowly apply the juice to the cat's side, near the base of her tail, or on her hind leg. These areas should be relatively easy for the cat to reach. Rub the juice into her fur so it doesn't drip off her body.

3. The cat will lick off the juice, thereby ingesting it. If your cat has long hair, consider brushing her before you apply the Noni. This way she will be less likely to ingest excessive hair when she washes off the Noni.

## SERVING GUIDELINES FOR CATS:

- For injuries, apply Noni directly on the wound. Also give your cat as much as one tablespoonful of Noni two or three times a day. Apply it to her fur or inject it directly into her mouth.
- For chronic conditions, try one or two teaspoonfuls of Noni, two or three times a day.
- For serious or life-threatening conditions, try giving two teaspoonfuls, four to eight times a day. When cats are this ill, it is better to insert the Noni directly into their mouth with an eyedropper or plastic syringe. When they start to object, you'll know they are feeling better.
- For trauma, and both before and after surgery, give a one-ounce serving. This will help speed recovery. During recovery, you can also give one teaspoonful every few hours.

- Continue until the condition improves, then reduce or discontinue the serving.
- A single one-ounce serving can sometimes be all that is needed for relatively minor health conditions.
- A feline Maintenance Serving would be about one-half to one teaspoonful a day.

Amounts for animals are usually measured in CCs. Your plastic syringe tube may therefore list only CCs.
Here are the equivalents:

| One teaspoonful = 5 CCs. |
| --- |
| One tablespoonful = 15 CCs. |
| One ounce = 30 CCs. |

## TIPS FOR GIVING NONI TO DOGS:

You could give your dog a Maintenance Serving in his food and he probably won't even notice. But when using Noni to alleviate health conditions, it is better to take Noni on an empty stomach either by itself or with water.

Before trying creative ways to give Noni fruit juice to your dog, pour the serving into his empty food bowl and see if he will lap it up. (It doesn't hurt to try.) If this doesn't work, try putting the Noni in a bowl with an amount of water that he will drink at one time. It is best to do this when he is thirsty. If that doesn't work either, you will have to insert the Noni directly into his mouth using a plastic syringe tube. Here's how:

Fill a large plastic syringe tube with the amount of Noni fruit juice you want to give your dog. You can find large plastic syringe tubes, which can hold up to two ounces of liquid, in pet stores that specialize in parrots. These large syringe tubes are used to hand feed baby macaws.

Have your dog sit.

Position yourself beside your dog's right shoulder (assuming you are right-handed). Stand or kneel, depending on your dog's size. Hold the syringe in your right hand. Show him the syringe and let him sniff it. Give him lots of pats and praise.

1. Wrap your left arm around your dog's shoulder and slide your left hand under his chin. Gently lift his chin, so he is looking up. He may respond by kissing you.

2. Insert the end of the syringe tube inside the back corner of his cheek. Use either the right or left side of his face, whichever side is easiest for you. The end of the syringe should be pointing down, between the inside of his cheek and his teeth. Your left hand should be underneath his lower jaw, gently keeping his chin pointed towards the ceiling. You don't need to open his mouth as you will be inserting the Noni inside his cheek and not between his teeth.

3. Squeeze the juice inside his cheek as fast as he will drink it. He will use his tongue to lap it up. The trick is to keep his nose pointing up, the syringe pointing down and to work quickly. Reassure him by talking to him constantly and looking kindly in his eyes. Have patience and always praise. Sooner or later, you will be able to give him Noni fruit juice without spilling a drop—or maybe only one or two.

## SERVING GUIDELINES FOR DOGS:

Evaluate your dog's condition as you might evaluate your own and select from the drinking applications in this book. You may need to modify the procedures to suit him and some just won't work for pets. (Can you imagine your dog doing the Noni

Gargle?) Also try the Noni topical and internal applications that are appropriate for your dog's condition.

- Dogs that weigh over one hundred pounds can receive the same amounts, according to the same procedures, as adult humans.
- Give medium-size dogs the same amount as you would give children.
- Small dogs can receive the same amounts as you would give to cats.

# -53-

# Giving Noni to Horses

For horses and ponies, from backyard pets to racehorses.

## WHEN TO GIVE NONI TO HORSES:

- To enhance performance.
- To improve health and overall condition.
- To prepare for show and racing.
- To enhance recovery from illness, disease and injury.

## HOW TO GIVE NONI TO HORSES:

**Noni can be given to horses both orally and topically.**
- When giving Noni orally, it is best to give it without food, which is also true for humans. Fill a plastic syringe tube with the amount of Noni you wish to give. Insert the end of the syringe tube into the corner of the horse's mouth as if you were administering paste wormer, and squirt the Noni in.
- The second best method is to offer Noni in a small bowl. However, if the horse smacks her lips and tongue while savoring the taste of Noni, she can send drops of Noni flying in all directions. This can be messy and wasteful.
- If your horse cannot drink Noni politely from a bowl, you will have to add Noni to some grain. Or try mixing Noni with molasses.

## SERVING GUIDELINES FOR HORSES:

If your horse is healthy, start with one or two ounces of Noni daily. After a week—if you began with one ounce—increase the serving to two ounces a day as maintenance. You will know that your horse is getting too much Noni when his stools get loose or his energy and zest for life become more than you can handle. Then reduce the daily amount to one ounce. You might even have to stop giving him Noni for a day or two.

Performance horses and those in training may need as much as four to six ounces of Noni a day.

For illness or injury, start with a two-ounce serving. Administer a second two-ounce serving several hours later. Observe your horse's behavior carefully and adjust the amount of Noni accordingly. For example, if she is feeling better, continue giving her two, two-ounce servings of Noni daily until her stools loosen or she becomes too zesty. If she is injured and needs to rest—but the Noni is making her too lively—reduce the oral servings and focus on topical applications.

If her condition does not seem to be improving, or improves slowly, continue to give two-ounce servings every few hours.

| | |
|---|---|
| 1 ounce = 2 tablespoonfuls = 30 cc = 30 ml | |
| 2 ounces = 4 tablespoonfuls = 60 cc = 60 ml | |

## HERE ARE SOME IDEAS FOR APPLYING NONI TOPICALLY TO HORSES:

- Mix equal parts of Noni fruit juice and skin lotion. Add some Noni seed oil if you have some. Massage into the area. This can be especially helpful for tight, stiff or overworked muscles.
- Mix Noni with a favorite liniment, and use as you would liniment.

- Try Noni-clay poultices (page 251). Noni Clay can hasten recovery, draw out toxins and normalize cells. Try it on swellings, sprains and internal injuries.
- Apply Noni fruit juice directly onto open wounds.
- Soak a cloth in Noni fruit juice and wrap the cloth around whatever part of the horse's leg requires attention. For relatively large areas, or for a more economical procedure, use a mixture of equal parts Noni and water.

## MORE ABOUT GIVING NONI TO HORSES:

If you consider that the average horse weighs about 1,204 to 1,500 pounds, almost ten times the weight of many adult people, you might think that horses would need about ten times the amount of Noni. But this is not so. In fact, horses seem to respond better to Noni than most people do. This may be because horses are naturally sensitive creatures, or because they do not harbor mindsets that can inhibit greater health. In fact, too much Noni can make horses feel too good, which can make them difficult to manage.

# -54-

# A Technique for
# Sharing Noni with Others

This method highlights the advantages of sharing Noni in a group environment.

## INVITE PEOPLE TO SHARE
## NONI IN A GROUP:

- When you would like to offer your friends a supportive environment when taking their First Serving.
- To give people a structured environment in which they can update their Noni Health Evaluation Sheet #2 (pages 22 and 23), their Noni Progress Chart (page 26) and their Noni Goal Achievement Chart (page 37).
- To boost everyone's confidence in Noni as they share each other's successes.
- To maximize the enthusiasm and excitement a group of people can feel when they share a common experience.

## HOW TO SHARE NONI WITH OTHERS:

**1. Create a comfortable environment.**
Invite your friends and associates to a special get-together where you will be sharing information about Noni and offering them a chance to try it. You will be planning something fun, interesting and informative that meets people's needs for health improvement, community, education, entertainment and support.

**2. Tell your Noni Story.**

Tell how you found out about Noni, how you took your
First Serving and the first health improvements that you
noticed. If you like, share your Noni Progress Chart and
your Noni Goal Achievement Chart, and let them see for
themselves how your symptoms have improved. If you
are involved in distributing Noni, talk about how you got
involved in this facet of Noni, too.

Invite one or two guests who are already taking Noni to
tell their Noni stories too. Keep stories brief and to the
point. They should build a feeling of anticipation among
guests who are new to Noni.

**3. Fill out the Noni evaluation charts.**

Pass around copies of the Health Evaluation Sheets,
Noni Progress Chart and Noni Goal Achievement Chart.
Explain how the charts can help them. Give people time
to fill out the charts.

This is a great opportunity for those who are already Noni
enthusiasts to re-evaluate their health and relay their
progress to the group. Some people may want to keep
their data private, and this desire should be respected.

**4. Talk about how to evaluate the Immediate Effects of
Noni.**

Show your guests the book, *101 Ways to Use Noni*, and
talk about how easy it is to take Noni and how versatile
Noni can be. Refer to Chapter 3, "Evaluating the
Immediate Effects of Noni." Explain that, when taking a
First Serving, we like to follow the procedure outlined in
this chapter because it is the best way for people to notice
Noni's effects as soon as possible. When people notice

positive effects right away, they will be more likely to see the long-term potential for improving their health with Noni.

Give people some time to fill out the Chart of Reference Points for Evaluating the Immediate Effects of Noni.

**5. Offer Noni to the group.**
Make this occasion special, even if most people in the group are already taking Noni. Bring in enough wine glasses for everyone. Measure and pour an ounce of Noni into each glass. Then invite everyone to drink their Noni—but one person at a time.

Before he or she drinks the Noni, remind the individual to put attention on his or her vision, lung capacity, and sense of calmness, vital energy, and well-being as described in Chapter 3. Ask everyone else to pay attention. The group will watch and lend support as each person takes a serving. The group will also try to notice anything different about the person afterwards. Some changes may be dramatic enough that almost anyone can see them, like a change in posture, complexion, facial expression and degree of relaxation. A few people might even be able to sense shifts in the person's energy after taking Noni.

After each individual takes a serving, ask what they are feeling. Let them describe how their eyesight and lung capacity and other reference points feel different. Ask the rest of the group to share the differences that they notice, too. Have the individual record his or her experiences in the Chart of Reference Points.

6. **Getting Started with Noni.**
   Explain how people can determine how much Noni to take each day. There are several approaches to doing this described in this book. Refer to The Easy Way to Select Your Noni Serving Size, on page 51. Also mention the procedures for Maintenance, plus Acute, Chronic and Serious Conditions.

   Talk about the ways to begin taking Noni: Gradually Introducing Noni to Your Diet (page 43) and the Loading Serving (page 47). Go around the room and ask each person how they started drinking Noni. If they are new to Noni, ask them how they think they might start.

   If you haven't already done so, pass around a copy of *101 Ways to Use Noni*. Discuss which procedure they might try first if they were drinking Noni regularly.

7. **Listen, answer questions, and offer the next step.**
   Ask if anyone has any questions or comments about Noni. Listen attentively to each question and answer as best you can. Listening is important because people's confidence grows if they know they are being heard.

   Finally, you want to tell everyone how they can get Noni on a regular basis. Some Noni distributors have trouble with this step because they don't want to feel as though they are "selling" something to their friends. Ideally, somebody will ask how to get more Noni, in which case you can tell them. (Or, beforehand, you can ask one of your close associates to ask this question in case nobody else does.)

# YOUR NONI STORY:

Ask yourself how Noni has helped you and your family. If Noni has helped you in any way, then you do indeed have a story to tell. Noni stories help people build an emotional connection to Noni. This is an essential key to sharing Noni with others. When someone has a heart connection to Noni, then conversations about Noni flow naturally.

Do not underestimate the importance of your Noni story. It is something you started to write the moment you heard about Noni, and you add a new chapter with each level of success that you achieve. Your Noni story is your legacy. It should inspire others when they hear it and yourself when you tell it.

# MORE ABOUT SHARING NONI WITH OTHERS:

This procedure provides an opportunity for people to discover Noni and to know within their heart if Noni is right for them. Without this heart connection, they won't be as committed to drinking Noni. Those who believe in Noni not only become good customers; they also have a story to tell, and therefore have all the requisites to becoming reliable, committed distributors.

This procedure is ideal for a group that consists of people new to Noni, plus those who are already Noni enthusiasts. However, you can modify these steps and follow them with only one or two other people to whom you are introducing Noni.

A big concern about introducing Noni to a group—or even to one person—is that they won't feel anything. Trust Noni and Trust Life. Sometimes it seems that Noni chooses people more than people choose Noni. Try not to be attached to the outcome of whether or not someone will feel Noni's effects immediately or not. Know that those people who are meant to feel attuned to Noni will be. All you can do is provide the optimal environment for positive results, which is what this procedure is designed to do.

If someone says, "I don't feel anything." Tell them, "Okay, let's wait a few minutes, let someone else have a turn, and then we'll check back with you." It may take a few minutes for that person's body to respond to Noni. Or it may take a few weeks.

There will always be people who ask the hard questions. They may be skeptical, but they are also willing to be convinced. After all, they did show up to learn more about Noni, didn't they? So they are not as closed-minded as they may sound. If Noni does indeed work for these people, they are likely to become loyal Noni enthusiasts.

Many people experience immediate effects after taking Noni. When they have the opportunity to experience these effects in a group—with all the support and community around them—the excitement for Noni can become unbelievable.

The steps in this procedure are designed to build enthusiasm for Noni. As these feelings grow during the evening, the more excited and open people will be. The less likely they will be to say "I don't feel anything," and the more likely they will be to say, "Wow, this Noni is fantastic!"

# -SECTION 2-

# TOPICAL APPLICATIONS

Noni topical applications are surprisingly versatile. Use them not only for skin conditions, but also to help the body heal, repair and detoxify organs and cells inside the body. Noni can do this because of its unusual ability to penetrate the skin, allowing the cells to transport Noni's beneficial compounds to areas that need them.

Drinking Noni fruit juice enhances the effects of Noni topical applications, so it is always a good idea to combine the two. From Section 1 of this book, select a procedure for drinking Noni that best suits your condition. Then choose the topical applications in Section 2 that would support your healing process.

Or, take another approach based on the principle that topical Noni applications draw to the affected area Noni beneficial compounds taken orally. Simply apply a topical Noni application where you want the beneficial compounds in your oral servings to go. Then drink your serving of Noni. This gives you some control as to where you want Noni to work.

As you read this section, you may notice that some ailments can be addressed by a few different applications. Try them all and likely one will work best and fit most conveniently into your lifestyle. When you try a Noni topical application, use it three times before judging how well you think it works.

A few of the topical applications in this Section employ special mixtures of Noni and water that I call "Dilutions." (For more about Noni Dilutions, see page 2.)

Topical Applications are also the answer when people are unable to drink Noni or when, as in the case of some children, they simply don't want to drink it.

This Section begins with a discussion of Noni Compresses and Poultices. These topical applications have the most versatile uses, so I listed them first for convenience.

# -55-

# The Noni Compress

Place a Noni Compress directly on the skin to help conditions inside the body. Apply it at room temperature or with an ice pack.

## USE A NONI COMPRESS FOR:

- Athletic injuries.
- Carpal tunnel syndrome.
- Injuries and conditions of the bones and joints.
- Injuries and conditions that require cold therapeutic applications.
- Painful areas.
- Sprains.
- Swelling and inflammation.
- To accelerate healing in areas where surgery has occurred.
- Tumors.
- Women's labia after childbirth.
- And to strengthen joints to prevent injuries.

## HOW TO MAKE AND APPLY
## A NONI COMPRESS:

1. Select a compress pad large enough to cover the affected area. (Read more about compress pads on page 227.)

2.  Refer to the information box on page 228 to select the amount of Noni you will need for the size of the compress pad you have chosen. Pour this amount of Noni into a bowl.

3.  Place the pad in the bowl and gently press down on the pad to help it soak up all the Noni. The side that is facing down will have a layer of pulp on it.

4.  When you remove the pad from the bowl, wipe up any pulp that remains in the bowl using the pulpy side of the pad.

5.  Center the wet pad over the affected area. The pulpy side should be touching the skin. The Compress will feel cold.

    **Optional:** Cover the Compress with plastic wrap and then with an old hand towel to prevent your clothing from being stained by any Noni that may drip. The plastic also keeps the compress moist and warm.

## MORE ABOUT THE NONI COMPRESS:

Keep the Compress in place for at least half an hour. Apply the Compress once or twice a day (or each night before bed), until the condition improves. If you need a cold application such as for sprains, wrap an ice pack in a thin towel and place it over the Compress.

If you want to move around while wearing the Compress, secure it to your body. Use whatever material you think would work best on the area. For example, try using gauze bandage, first-aid tape, an ace bandage, a towel or a bandanna. Be sure not to tie the Compress on too tightly.

If you need a heated topical application, try a Noni Poultice as described in the following chapter. Applying heat to a topical application encourages Noni's beneficial compounds to be absorbed into the body and is not suggested for Noni Compresses. Compresses consist of undiluted Noni, which contains a relatively high concentration of beneficial compounds. Heat can cause too many beneficial compounds to enter the body too quickly, which can irritate the skin and initiate a release of toxins. This can cause a rash or a cleansing reaction (see page 410). If a skin rash or pimples erupt after using a Noni Compress, drink more purified water to help flush the toxins through the kidneys instead.

If you would simply like to warm the Noni Compress to make it more comfortable, see Ways to Warm Noni on page 405.

## ABOUT COMPRESS PADS
## (AND POULTICE PADS):

**Use can use several kinds of pads:**
- Gauze pads come in convenient sizes and are sterile, which is important if the skin is wounded. Do not unfold a gauze pad in order to cover a larger area. The pad should be several layers thick to hold enough Noni. Use two pads side-by-side if necessary.
- Paper towels make excellent compress pads. They are more economical than gauze pads and most people have them readily available. Fold paper towels in half twice so they are four layers thick.
- You could also use cheesecloth, but it has to be folded several times and can be awkward to work with.
- To make rolled gauze into a compress pad, unroll the gauze and then fold it several times to an appropriate size and thickness.
- Use paper napkins to cover relatively large areas.

## GUIDELINES FOR HOW MUCH LIQUID TO USE WITH VARIOUS SIZES OF COMPRESS PADS AND POULTICE PADS:

| | |
|---|---|
| One 2" x 2" gauze pad | One-half tablespoonful |
| One 4" x 4" gauze pad | One tablespoonful |
| One paper towel folded in quarters | One tablespoonful |
| Three paper napkins sandwiched together | One ounce |

**Note:** These amounts may vary depending on the thickness and absorbency of the material used.

# -56-

# The Noni Poultice

Make Noni Poultices with a mixture of Noni fruit juice and water. Apply Noni Poultices at room temperature or heated.

## USE A NONI POULTICE FOR:

- Conditions that involve the internal organs.
- Conditions that require a heated application.
- Asthma, bronchitis and other lung conditions.
- Diabetes (when placed over the pancreas).
- Endometriosis.
- Kidney and adrenal problems.
- Liver complaints.
- Mastitis.
- Menstrual cramps.
- Old injuries not completely healed (heat plus the penetrating effects of the Noni Poultice can bring Noni beneficial compounds to the cells that need them).
- Painful areas.
- Sluggish or malfunctioning organs.

## HOW TO MAKE A NONI POULTICE:

1. Select a poultice pad large enough to cover the affected area. (Read about poultice pads on page 227.)

2. Refer to the information box on page 228 to select the amount of liquid you will need for the size of the poultice

pad you have chosen. Half of this amount will be Noni, and half will be purified water.

3. Pour the amount of Noni fruit juice you will need into a bowl. Measure an equal amount of purified water.

4. Swirl the bowl so the Noni is moving in a circular direction. Keep swirling as your pour the water into the Noni in a steady, uninterrupted stream. Continue to swirl the bowl for another few seconds to mix the liquids together. You have now made a 1:1 Dilution of Noni.

## HOW APPLY A NONI POULTICE:

1. Place the poultice pad on the 1:1 Dilution and gently press down on the pad to help it soak up all the liquid.

2. When you remove the pad from the bowl, wipe up any pulp that remains in the bowl using the pulpy side of the pad.

3. Center the wet pad over the affected area. The pulpy side should be touching the skin.

   **Optional:** Cover the Poultice first with plastic wrap, then with an old hand-towel to protect your clothing from any Noni that may drip. The plastic also keeps the Poultice moist and warm.

## MORE ABOUT NONI POULTICES:

Keep the Poultice in place for at least half an hour or overnight. Apply the Poultice once or twice a day (or each night before bed), until the condition improves.

Poultices can be applied hot to encourage Noni's beneficial

compounds to be absorbed into the body. See page 233 for "Ways to Heat Noni Poultices."

If you want to move around while wearing the Poultice, secure the Poultice to your body. Use whatever material you think will work best for the area. Try using a gauze bandage, first-aid tape, an ace bandage, a towel or a bandanna. Be sure not to tie the Poultice on too tightly.

Noni Poultices consist of a 1:1 Dilution. This Dilution is made with equal amounts of Noni fruit juice and water, combined in a special way that activates Noni's restorative energies. These restorative energies add to the benefits of Noni's beneficial compounds. In this case, the added water also provides a pathway for Noni's compounds to penetrate the body.

Use only distilled water, spring water, purified tap water or untreated well water when making Noni Poultices. Chlorine, fluorine, and other chemicals used to treat tap water can interfere with the body's ability to absorb and use Noni's beneficial compounds.

## HOW NONI COMPRESSES
## AND POULTICES ARE DIFFERENT:

- Compresses are made of Noni fruit juice alone. Poultices contain equal parts of Noni and water.
- Compresses have a greater tendency to draw out toxins. This is a natural effect of a topical application of undiluted Noni fruit juice. Poultices are made with a Noni dilution that employs one of Noni's restorative energies. In poultice form, this dilution encourages Noni's beneficial compounds to move more deeply into the body.
- Compresses are preferred for joint and bone conditions. The restorative energies of undiluted Noni have an affinity with structural components of the body, including joints and bones on a macro level, and protein molecules on a micro level. Poultices are preferred for organ conditions

because the restorative energy of the 1:1 Dilution encourages cells and organs to interact in a more healthy way with each other, with their local environment, as well as with the rest of the body. Poor interactions in these areas are a primary cause for disease.

- Compresses are applied at room temperature or chilled with ice. The body may not be able to handle in balance the sped-up detoxification that a heated compress could produce. Poultices may be applied at room temperature or heated. Heat complements the penetrating effect of the 1:1 Dilution. Cold would work against it.

## HOW COMPRESSES
## AND POULTICES ARE SIMILAR:

- Both may be used for pain.
- Both may accelerate healing and improve flexibility and circulation in the affected area.
- Both soften the skin on which they are placed.
- Both may be placed over areas where the skin has been cut, scraped or bruised, or that has a rash or other skin condition, but neither is meant specifically for skin conditions. For skin conditions, refer to the Noni Astringent and After-shave (page 243), The Noni Rash Plaster (page 325), or the Noni Topical Splash (page 335).

## SHOULD I USE A NONI
## COMPRESS OR POULTICE?

If you are not sure which to use, ask yourself:

- Is the target area related to a bone, joint, muscle or ligament? If so, use a Compress.

- Does the target area involve soft tissue or an internal organ? If so, use a Poultice.
- Would the target area benefit from a cold application? If so, use a Compress.
- Would the area feel better with heat? If so, use a Poultice.
- Does the ailment in the target area involve toxicity, swelling or pus? If so, use a Compress.

## WAYS TO HEAT NONI POULTICES:

**METHOD #1**
Follow the instructions for making Noni Poultices using purified, heated water. This method won't make the poultice hot, but it will take the chill off.

**METHOD #2**
This method will make a Noni Poultice as warm as you can get it, without compromising Noni's beneficial compounds.

1. Find two glass or stainless steel pots. (Do not use aluminum pots.) One pot should be able to fit inside the other.

2. Fill the larger pot with water and bring the water to a boil. Then take the pot off the heat.

3. Prepare the Noni-water mixture you will use for the Noni Poultice. Pour the Noni-water into the smaller pot.

4. Put the bottom of the smaller pot into the pot with the hot water. Make sure none of the heated water seeps into the Noni-water mixture in the smaller pot.

5. Stir the Noni-water mixture with your finger. When the liquid gets too hot to touch, remove the pot from the hot water.

6. Lay the poultice pad on the Noni-water in the small pot. Before you place the Poultice on the body, retest its temperature to make sure it won't be too hot for the area of the body where the Poultice will be placed.

## METHOD #3

Use this heating method when you want to add heat to an application, and for the heat to last as long as possible.

1. Bring a large pot of water to a simmer. Immerse a large folded towel into the heated water. The thicker the towel, the longer it will retain heat. Wear rubber gloves for protection and wring out the towel.

2. Place the Noni Poultice on the body. The Poultice will feel cold on contact, but it will heat up immediately once you apply the hot towel, as follows.

3. Test the towel's temperature to make sure it won't be too hot for the person receiving it. If so, let it cool for a few minutes before applying, or put a dry towel between the Poultice and the heated towel.

4. Place the hot towel over the Poultice. When the towel cools, you can reheat it and reapply it without removing the Poultice.

# -57-

# Noni Abdominal Conditioner

Use this procedure to alleviate certain symptoms or as part of your health maintenance and improvement program.

## USE THE NONI
## ABDOMINAL CONDITIONER TO:

- Alleviate and prevent constipation and intestinal blockages.
- Alleviate intestinal inflammation.
- Alleviate fever.
- Improve the movement of matter through the intestines.
- Improve the general health of organs located in the affected area, including the intestines, stomach, pancreas, liver, gallbladder, spleen and bladder (and for women, the ovaries and uterus).
- Increase circulation to these organs.
- Stimulate the "dantien," which, according to Chinese Medicine, is the source and powerhouse of energy in the body.

## HOW TO MAKE THE NONI-LOTION
## MIXTURE FOR THIS PROCEDURE:

1. Turn a bottle of Noni upside down then right side up a few times to mix the Noni pulp throughout the juice.

2. Measure one teaspoonful of Noni and pour it into a medicine cup.

3. Use the same measuring spoon to measure one-half to one teaspoonful of your favorite body lotion.

4. Use a cotton swab to wipe the body lotion from the teaspoon into the medicine cup that contains the Noni. Use the same swab to mix the lotion and Noni juice together. Mix well. The mixture will be liquid.

## HOW TO APPLY THE NONI ABDOMINAL CONDITIONER:

1. Bring the Noni-lotion mixture, as well as the cotton swab you used to make it, to your bedroom.

2. Remove the clothing from your ribcage down to your pubic bone, and lie down on your back.

3. Use the cotton swab to pour a portion of the Noni mixture onto your abdomen.

4. Use both hands to massage the Noni mixture over your entire abdomen. Massage both sides of your belly, from under your ribs down to your pubic bone. Apply more of the Noni-lotion mixture if your abdomen starts to feel dry.

5. After about five minutes, use a tissue to wipe off any excess Noni-lotion mixture. Replace your clothing. By now, the Noni will be soaked into your skin and shouldn't stain.

# MORE ABOUT THE NONI ABDOMINAL CONDITIONER:

Cover your abdomen generously with the Noni-lotion mixture. After you do this procedure once, you will have a better idea of exactly how much Noni-lotion you need. Then adjust how much you make next time.

Apply daily until symptoms abate, or several times a day if you are applying it for fever. (See also the Noni for the Immune System on page 305.) For general health maintenance and improvement, use the Noni Abdominal Conditioner at least once or twice a week. The technique is most effective when done lying down as your abdominal muscles are then relaxed. This way, it is easier to access your internal organs. I find it most convenient to do this procedure before going to sleep at night.

During the massage, you may find pockets of gas, intestinal blockages and painful areas that you didn't know you had. Most people will have a few tender spots. Use common sense and work gently on these areas. Avoid painful areas if the massage makes them feel worse. See a doctor if you are concerned about any lumps or painful areas that you might find.

Many people suffer from a variety of intestinal conditions including constipation, flatulence, pain, inflammation, yeast and parasites. These conditions—no matter what their cause—inhibit the amount of life-giving energy naturally moving through the abdomen. As a result, other internal organs such as the stomach, pancreas, liver, spleen, bladder, gall bladder and reproductive organs may suffer.

As body lotion soaks into the skin, which it is designed to do, Noni's beneficial compounds will soak in along with it. Thus, the Noni Abdominal Conditioner brings Noni's beneficial compounds directly to the internal organs. These compounds have proven effective against inflammation, parasites, yeast and bacteria.[20] They also enhance the absorption of nutrients and help the body cleanse and purify itself. Noni's anti-inflammatory properties are soothing to many abdominal conditions that involve inflammation.

After a few applications, you may notice improvements in your bowel regularity. You will find fewer gas pockets, and any tender spots you might have should abate or just go away. If you find yourself going to the bathroom more often, stop the treatment for a while. Your body should normalize within a few days.

The Noni Abdominal Conditioner is an excellent addition to any weight-loss program. The procedure requires people to touch and massage an area of their body that they may harbor negative thoughts and feelings about due to excess fat. Use the time spent during the massage to nurture positive thoughts and feelings. For example, repeat a positive statement or affirmation such as "I love my body. I am grateful for my body and the work my organs do."

You can also use Intention and repeat a statement that you would like to manifest into a reality, such as, "I am slender, fit and healthy." Say these words as sincerely as possible and believe them. Eventually, you will form a new concept of yourself, which "as above, so below" can be reflected in your outer world.

Repeat these affirmations to yourself silently or aloud while you do the Noni Abdominal Conditioner each day. (See Using Intention with Noni on page 115).

---

[20] *Noni—Polynesia's Natural Pharmacy* (Vineyard: Pride Publishing, 1997), pp. 6, 7, 17, 18.

# HERE ARE SOME WAYS
# TO MASSAGE YOUR ABDOMEN:

- Use large sweeping clockwise circles. (Clockwise looking down at your body.) This is the direction that material travels through your large intestine.
- Work your abdomen in a kneading motion.
- Press your fingertips deeply into your belly and make small circles with your fingertips. Do this at several different points on your abdomen, particularly where you feel intestinal blockages or gas pockets. Be gentle over points of pain.
- Use your knuckles and press into your abdomen making circles.
- Rub under your ribcage on both sides of your body, but particularly your right side where your liver is located.
- Hold your hands on your hips with your fingers pointing towards each other. Your fingers should be in front of your hips and your thumbs in back. Press your fingertips into your abdomen. Massage by bending and straightening your fingers. Then, with your thumbs still holding your hips, keep moving your fingers in this way as you point them lower toward your feet, and then upward toward your ribcage and then back down again.
- Spend some time massaging the dantien, which is located in the middle of the abdomen just below the belly button. Stimulating this area, and especially breathing into it, can increase the flow of energy throughout the body, giving you life, health, and strength.

# -58-

# A Noni Procedure
# for Ailing Joints

A way for painful areas to absorb and benefit from concentrated Noni beneficial compounds.

## TRY THIS PROCEDURE FOR:

Pain in the hands, knuckles, fingers, wrists, elbows, neck, knees, ankles, and toes due to conditions such as:

- Arthritis.
- Bursitis.
- Fibromyalgia.
- Injuries.
- Neuralgia.
- Sprains.
- Stiffness.

Also try this procedure to strengthen joints such as knees and ankles before exercise to help avoid injury.

## HOW TO DO THE NONI
## PROCEDURE FOR AILING JOINTS:

1. Refer to page 318 to make a recipe of Noni Paste.

2. Measure a one-quarter teaspoonful of Noni Paste. Use a cotton swab to remove it from the measuring spoon and put it into a medicine cup or other small container.

3.  Measure a one-quarter teaspoonful of your favorite skin lotion. Use the same cotton swab to wipe the lotion off the measuring spoon and into the Noni Paste.

4.  Mix the Noni Paste and the lotion together.

5.  Spread the Noni Paste-lotion mixture on the area to be treated. Rub it in until all that remains is some remnants of Noni pulp. Use a paper towel to brush these remnants off your skin. Your skin will feel a little sticky until the Paste-lotion completely dries.

6.  Make another batch if you want to add more Paste-lotion to the area or if you want to treat the opposite joint.

## MORE ABOUT THE
## NONI PROCEDURE FOR AILING JOINTS:

Noni Paste mixes easily with skin lotion and absorbs surprisingly well. After you brush off the dried Noni pulp, you won't be able to see the application on your skin, so you won't have to wash it off.

This procedure brings a concentration of Noni beneficial compounds to an ailing area. These compounds include agents that help with pain, inflammation and cell regeneration, which can be particularly beneficial for joint conditions. After one application, you should notice a difference in the way the area feels. Flexibility and use of the joint should improve after repeated applications. As a side benefit, your skin should feel softer and healthier as Noni brings essential nutrients to the cells.

Repeat this procedure one or more times a day for as long as needed.

# -59-

## Noni Astringent
## and After-shave

An astringent draws together or constricts body tissues and is effective for stopping the flow of blood or other secretions.

### USE NONI ASTRINGENT AND AFTER-SHAVE:

- As you would regular after-shave: on the face, legs or underarms.
- For skin that gets irritated or dry from shaving, allergies or other reasons.
- As a first aid application for abrasions, cuts, scrapes and other minor wounds.
- For burns and scalds.
- For sunburn.
- For widespread skin eruptions and inflamed skin.

### HOW TO MAKE NONI
### ASTRINGENT AND AFTER-SHAVE:

This procedure combines Noni fruit juice with the popular witch hazel astringent cleanser, which contains approximately fourteen percent alcohol, witch hazel distillate, and witch hazel extract.[21]

1. Obtain an empty four-ounce plastic bottle from the drug store. Such bottles are commonly used to transport shampoo or hand lotion.

---

[21] I use Dickinson's® 104% All Natural Botanical Witch Hazel Formula.

2.  Pour one tablespoonful of Noni fruit juice into the bottle.

3.  Pour four tablespoonfuls (two ounces) of witch hazel into the bottle. The bottle will be a little more than half-full.

4.  Put the lid on the bottle and gently shake the bottle to mix the two ingredients together.

## HOW TO APPLY NONI ASTRINGENT AND AFTER-SHAVE:

1.  Apply the Noni Astringent and After-shave to your skin with a cotton ball or with your hands.

2.  Allow the liquid to air dry on your skin. Apply additional Noni Astringent as needed.

## MORE ABOUT NONI ASTRINGENT AND AFTER-SHAVE:

Don't shake the bottle of Noni fruit juice before pouring the Noni. The more watery part of the juice, found at the top of a Noni bottle, is better because it is less pulpy.

Except in hot climates, you can leave Noni Astringent and After-shave at room temperature for a few days. Otherwise, store it in the refrigerator for your next use.

If you have been nicked by the razor blade, apply extra Noni Astringent and After-shave to the cut. Both Noni and witch hazel can help stop bleeding. Because this formula contains witch hazel, avoid contact with the eyes.

Witch hazel is a medicinal herb whose distilled extract can be found in most drug stores or health food stores. Witch hazel has been used by the North American Indians as poultices for painful swellings and tumors. It is also helpful for bruises, inflammatory swellings, insect bites, burns, scalds, varicose veins, dermatitis, and to help stop bleeding.[22]

Noni Astringent and After-shave also helps to soften and smooth the skin, and can relieve dry, chapped skin, pimples and wrinkles.

---

[22] Mrs. M. Grieve, *A Modern Herbal, Volume II,* (New York, NY: Dover Publications), 1971, page 851.

# -60-

## The Noni Back Compress

The Noni Back Compress consists of enough compress pads to cover the entire spine.

## A NONI BACK COMPRESS MAY BE HELPFUL FOR A VARIETY OF BACK CONDITIONS, INCLUDING:

- Backache.
- Broken ribs.
- Low back pain.
- Muscle spasms.
- Pinched nerves.
- Sore hips.
- Spinal weakness.
- Stress.
- Subluxation (dislocation of a vertebra).

## HOW TO MAKE AND APPLY A NONI BACK COMPRESS:

1. Regular 6" x 6" paper napkins are convenient and economical compress pads for this technique. Most adults will require five or six to cover the spine from the neck to the sacrum. Children may need three or four.

2. Warm the Noni:
   a. Fill a glass bowl with hot tap water.
   b. Fill a small plastic sandwich bag with one ounce of Noni fruit juice.
   c. Twist the open end of the bag so the Noni does not spill out. Hold the bag upright and submerge the end of the bag that contains the Noni under the hot water. Jiggle the bag so the heat disperses through the Noni.

3. Set the bag of Noni aside, empty the bowl of water and dry the bowl. Now pour the heated Noni into the bowl, which should still be warm from the hot water it once contained.

4. Have the person who is to receive the Noni Back Compress lay on his or her stomach with their back bare. Have them lay on a towel just in case any Noni drips off the back.

5. Bring the bowl of Noni and a pile of napkins with you to the person's bedside. (Use the extra napkins to wipe up any Noni that may spill or drip.)

6. Hold the edges of a napkin and press the center of the napkin into the bowl of Noni for a few seconds to absorb some of the Noni. Remove the napkin from the bowl and place the pulpy side of it on the sacrum, which is the lower end of the spine.

7. Press the center of another napkin into the bowl of Noni for a few seconds to absorb some of the liquid. Place this napkin, pulpy side down, next to the other napkin and higher up on the spine.

8. Repeat Step 7 until you have all the napkins placed along the spine. You may have some Noni left over in the bowl. If you do, remove the napkin on the area of the spine that is most troublesome, and put it back into the bowl to soak up more Noni. Wipe up any pulp that remains. Return the napkin to its previous location on the spine. You may have enough Noni left over to add a bit more to each of the other napkins as well.

## MORE ABOUT THE NONI
## BACK COMPRESS:

Leave the napkins in place for at least fifteen minutes. If the person on whom you are applying the compress falls asleep or wants to rest longer, leave the napkins in place until the individual wants to get up.

If the person feels cold, cover their back with an old towel. Or cover the napkins first with a sheet of plastic wrap and then cover the individual with a blanket.

When the application is finished, remove the napkins and toss them in the trash. Use extra dry napkins to wipe off any Noni that remains on the person's back.

Apply the Noni Back Compress at least once a day. Even after the pain goes away, continue daily applications for a few days to help avoid relapse.

The philosophy behind this procedure is if only one section of an organ ails, really the entire organ is not well. In other words, if your back hurts in one place, why not improve the condition of the entire spine? If you can uplift the health of the entire spine, you will be more likely to see improvement in the one area that is in pain. Likewise, if you uplift the health of the entire body, such as by drinking a daily serving of Noni, you will be improving the health of isolated ailing parts as well.

Another reason to apply the compress to the entire spine is that other areas of the spine tend to compensate and adapt for areas of pain and subluxation. These compensations may go unnoticed but they further weaken certain parts of the spine and misalign the posture. Treating the entire spine can strengthen these weaknesses. It can improve cellular communication throughout the spine, and help the spine function as a unified structure of the body.

**Optional:** Before the procedure, you may gently massage the back for a few minutes. Do so only if massage does not cause additional discomfort. Massage will increase circulation to the area to enhance the absorption of Noni's beneficial compounds.

To help with the pain, take a Noni Trauma Serving (page 95) before the Back Compress is applied.

# -61-
## Noni Clay

This is like a biological sponge for pain, toxins and malaise.

### TRY MIXING NONI WITH CLAY FOR:

- Abscesses.
- Arthritis.
- Conditions associated with congestion and toxins.
- Fever.
- Headaches.
- Heavy metal poisoning.
- Injuries.
- Lung conditions.
- Rheumatism.
- Swelling.
- Tumors.
- Sinusitis.

And when you want to access and release the emotional energy attached to local conditions.

### HOW TO MIX NONI WITH CLAY:

1. Measure one part of powdered clay and put it into a bowl.

2. Add one part purified water.

3. Add one part Noni fruit juice.

4. Mix the ingredients together into a paste using a non-metal spoon.

# MORE ABOUT MIXING NONI WITH CLAY:

Before measuring the Noni, turn the Noni bottle upside down then right side up a few times to mix the pulp with the watery portion of the juice.

How much is "one part" of each of the above ingredients can vary from one tablespoonful to several ounces. It depends on the size of the affected area. Noni-clay mixtures should completely cover the affected area.

In addition, the deeper inside the body the condition lays and the more serious the condition, the thicker the Noni-clay application should be. As a guideline: Cover areas that are relatively small (two inches or less in diameter), with a layer of Noni-clay one-eighth inch thick. Larger areas should have a layer at least one-quarter inch thick.

Several kinds of dried clay are available in health food stores. Choose the least expensive. You can also buy dried clay from ceramics supplies stores. Ask for "virgin" clay—clay that has not undergone any treatment since it was extracted from the quarry.

Use a plastic or wooden spoon to mix the Noni and clay. Metal can interfere with the charged particles in the clay, thus making the procedure less effective.[23]

# HOW TO APPLY NONI-CLAY:

1. Identify the affected area.

2. Cut a single layer of cheesecloth large enough to cover the chosen area, plus about four inches. Center it on the affected area. (You can also use a piece of gauze, unfolded to a single layer.)

---

[23] Raymond Dextreit and Michel Abehsera, *Our Earth Our Cure* (New York: Swan House Publishing, 1979), p. 17.

3. Using a wooden spoon, spread enough Noni-clay mixture over the cheesecloth to cover the chosen area to the thickness suggested above. There should be about two inches of cheesecloth leftover around all the edges. Use the back of the spoon to smooth the Noni-clay to a relatively even thickness.

4. Cover the Noni-clay with another layer or two of cheesecloth.

5. When you are finished, remove the Noni-clay by lifting the cheesecloth. Throw it in the trash. Wipe up the Noni-clay that remains on the area with a damp cloth.

## MORE ABOUT USING NONI-CLAY MIXTURES:

The cheesecloth allows you to remove the Noni-clay quickly and with minimal minimum of cleanup. This may be especially helpful for children or when alternating Noni-clay placement locations. Since wet Noni clay seeps through the cheesecloth, a single layer of it shouldn't reduce the procedure's beneficial effects.

If you do not have cheesecloth or gauze available, place the Noni-clay directly on the skin. However, it will be more difficult to remove when the procedure is over. Try using the side of a metal spoon to scrape off the Noni-clay then showering to remove it completely.

If rashes, skin eruptions, or itching occur during a Noni-clay application, remove the Noni-clay. These effects are likely the result of toxins the clay pulls from inside the body.

Leave Noni-clay applications in place at least one-half hour, though they could remain as long as two to four hours, or applied before bed and removed in the morning. Daily applications are recommended. But, if Noni-clay eases pain, it can be applied more frequently.

If you wish to keep the Noni-clay in place overnight, you will need to cover it with plastic wrap to protect your linens. However, if you are applying the Noni-clay in order to draw toxins from the body, it is better to keep the Noni-clay uncovered. The process of drawing out toxins and excesses from the body seems to correlate with the clay drying out. For pain and injuries, I have found the clay works just as well covered or uncovered.

Clay poultices are known for their ability to draw toxins from the body. Adding Noni to the clay lends "intelligence" to this process that regulates it and makes the release more harmonious and soothing. Adding Noni also releases the emotional energy associated with the condition. This doesn't usually happen when using clay alone. With Noni, cycles of toxin release and emotional release may alternate.

Unresolved emotions are often associated with disease or the original trauma of slow-healing injuries. Noni-clay can help release these old, pent-up emotions. Don't be surprised if you start to feel some of them.

In some way, emotions are usually involved in all our pains and illnesses. If the emotions are not resolved or put to ease as the condition heals, then recovery can be inhibited. During the emotional-release cycle, try to remember that these are old emotions coming forward. Although they may feel very "real," they are not necessarily real in present time. So try to be as objective about them as possible. Cry your heart out if you need to, but cry only for as long as you have to. Take the first window given to stop. Crying likes to perpetuate itself. During the process of crying, a moment comes when we have finished crying about a particular thing. Then we have a choice to stop crying. But the heart likes to take advantage of the release, and usually finds something else to cry about, so we start to cry for a different reason.

If you think the Noni-clay has stimulated a release of an old emotion, keep the crying focused on that one emotion. Give yourself permission to stop crying as soon as you no longer feel that one emotion. If several old emotions surface, be careful to let each one go as soon as the release finally occurs and the crying cycle stops. You will know when this occurs because you will feel emotionally spent, a sense of relief, a sense of inner peace, or your outlook on life will improve.

It is also possible to release emotions without having to process them through crying. If you would like to try this, here is a technique that might help: When you feel an emotion swell up inside, imagine it is contained inside soap bubbles. As the bubbles rise up, they pass out of your body. Imagine them floating upwards into the sky. Because the bubbles encase the emotion, they protect you from having to feel the full force of that emotion. If you try this technique, it helps to keep a notepad with you. As emotions arise, write down each one as you sense it bubbling up. See how long a list you can make. You may notice several flavors of a particular emotion, so use adjectives freely when you make your list. For example, you might write, "deep sadness, gut-wrenching sadness, bittersweet sadness, mild sadness," etc. Watch how emotions can alternate or repeat themselves. Each time a certain one comes up you may be releasing it at a deeper level. Writing down these emotions also allows you to identify them, to forgive the circumstances and people involved, and then to move on. When you can do this, cross the emotion off your list. Doing so symbolizes its release.

# HERE ARE SOME SUGGESTIONS FOR SPECIFIC NONI-CLAY APPLICATIONS:

- For headaches, apply Noni-clay alternately to the nape of the neck and then the forehead,[24] ten minutes at each placement, for a total of about one hour or until the pain is gone.
- For fevers, apply Noni-clay to the lower abdomen using Method #2. Remove the clay when it becomes warm.[25]
- For conditions such as arthritis and gout, apply Noni-clay to the afflicted areas to draw out the toxins and metabolic wastes that have pooled around the joints causing inflammation and pain.
- To help rid the mouth of mercury and other heavy metals, spread Noni-clay on the jaws. This will also serve as a Noni facial, and do wonders for your skin. Follow with a favorite moisturizer.
- For sinusitis, try Noni-clay on the forehead and upper cheeks. Also, apply Noni-clay over the liver. A congested liver is often associated with sinus conditions.

---

[24] Dextreit and Abehsera, p. 22.
[25] Ibid. p. 20.

# -62-
## Noni Cuticle Care

This procedure requires a batch of Noni Paste.

### USE NONI CUTICLE CARE FOR:

- Unhealthy, dry, overgrown or unsightly cuticles
- Injured cuticles or nails.
- Nail fungus.
- Nail infections.
- Painful cuticles or nails.

### HOW TO DO NONI CUTICLE CARE:

1. Prepare a batch of Noni Paste (page 318).

2. Use your fingertip or a cotton swab to spread a relatively thick layer of Noni Paste over the affected cuticles.

3. Cover the Noni Paste with an adhesive bandage.

## MORE ABOUT NONI CUTICLE CARE:

Leave the Noni Paste in place for as long as possible; though replace it and the adhesive bandage once or twice a day. Keep applying Noni Paste to the affected area until it heals and is pain-free.

Noni Paste contains a concentration of Noni beneficial compounds. As they absorb into your finger, it may tingle or feel warm. It may also make your hand feel more relaxed.

This procedure is much stronger than the Noni Nail Treatment because it employs Noni Paste. However, Noni Paste can take a day or two to make. While you are waiting, use the Noni Nail Treatment (page 315).

# -63-
# Easy Noni Skin Conditioner

A quick and easy way to improve the health of your skin.

## TRY THE EASY NONI
## SKIN CONDITIONER FOR:

- Daily skin-care maintenance on relatively small areas.
- Counteracting the effects of aging.
- Skin conditions of any kind that are relatively mild.
- Skin problems anywhere on your body.

## HOW TO APPLY THE
## EASY NONI SKIN CONDITIONER:

1. Pour your regular serving of Noni.

2. Drink all but a few drops.

3. Pour this leftover amount into the palm of your hand or pour it directly onto the skin that you want to treat.

4. Spread the Noni over the area.

# MORE ABOUT THE
# EASY NONI SKIN CONDITIONER:

The Easy Noni Skin Conditioner technique is worth mentioning because it is so very easy, takes only seconds to apply, and because the effects of Noni are so beneficial for the skin.

This technique is best suited for mild conditions. For more serious conditions try the Noni Rash Plaster on page 325, the Noni Poultice on page 229 or Noni Paste on page 317.

Using only a few drops of Noni should be a small enough amount that it shouldn't feel too sticky on your skin. If it does feel sticky, put a few drops of water on the skin where you have applied the Noni, rub it in, and let it air dry. Next time, add the water to the Noni before you apply it.

# -64-

# Noni to Enhance
# Dreams and Sleep

"I dream of Noni."

## TRY THIS TECHNIQUE TO:

- Enhance dream recall.
- Help you fall asleep at bedtime.

## HOW TO USE NONI TO
## ENHANCE SLEEP AND DREAMS:

1. Before you go to bed at night, prepare the following mixture of Noni and water, which is also called a 1:4 Dilution:
   a. Measure one tablespoonful of Noni fruit juice and pour it into a drinking glass.
   b. Use a one-cup measuring cup to measure two ounces (four tablespoonfuls) of purified water.
   c. Swirl the Noni by moving the glass in a circular motion. Keep swirling and add the water in a slow, steady, uninterrupted stream. Continue to swirl the mixture for a few more seconds to mix the liquids together.

2. Pour about a teaspoonful of the Dilution into a bowl.

3.  Make a poultice pad using half a cotton ball. Flatten the cotton by pulling on its edges.

4.  Put the cotton into the bowl of Noni. Bring the bowl and the glass of Dilution to your beside.

5.  When you are ready for bed, drink some (or all if you like) of the Noni-water mixture in the glass.

6.  Remove the cotton from the bowl and gently squeeze out excess liquid. It should be wet but not dripping wet.

7.  Place the flattened cotton in the center of your forehead, just above the bony ridge of your eyebrows. Gently press it against your forehead to help it adhere to your skin.

8.  Lay down on your back, close your eyes and focus on the relatively cool temperature of the Noni on your forehead. Pay attention to how the Noni warms with your body heat over time. This in itself can be very relaxing. Allow yourself to drift off to sleep.

## MORE ABOUT USING NONI TO ENHANCE SLEEP AND DREAMS:

You don't have to keep the cotton in place all night long. After it helps you fall asleep, it doesn't matter if it remains on your forehead or not. You could try keeping it there only for as long as you can lie comfortably on your back, and then remove it when you are ready to fall asleep. You may find, however, that the flat wet cotton will stay on your forehead even when you turn on your side. As the cotton dries, it will fall off. If you are concerned about it staining your pillow, put a towel underneath your head.

Mixing four parts of water with one part of Noni in the special way explained above releases one of Noni's restorative energies. This particular restorative energy brings harmony and balance to the nerves by improving communication throughout the nervous and sensory systems.

The area in the center of the forehead where you put the poultice pad is also called a "chakra." Chakras are centers of energy in the body. When a therapeutic substance is placed on the forehead chakra, it becomes a window to the brain and the therapeutic substance can affect brain function. When one places a poultice of a 1:4 Dilution there, the brain is soothed and relaxed. The pineal gland, located inside the brain, is encouraged to make melatonin, which is a substance that helps you fall asleep.

If drinking Noni tends to keep you awake at night, you may prefer to omit Step 5. However, the effects of a 1:4 Dilution are different from those of undiluted Noni because of the restorative energy brought forth. Drinking at least a few sips of the 1:4 Dilution before bed may promote sleep as it calms an over-stressed nervous system. (See also Using Noni as a Sleep Aid on page 169.)

The forehead chakra is also associated with the mind's eye and is referred to as the window to one's inner worlds or dream worlds. When a poultice of 1:4 Dilution is placed on a chakra center, it promotes balance and harmony in that chakra. This allows the chakra to open, or to open wider with greater strength and confidence if it has been somewhat closed. Since clear dream recall is often associated with an open forehead chakra, performing this technique can help you remember your dreams.

Many people like to remember their dreams because they have found that dreams are a source of truth. Through dreams, they can find answers, insights and guidance. If you would like to try to get an answer from your dreams, this simple technique may help:

1. Before bed, write down a question that you would like to receive insight about from your dreams. Copy the question several more times. This will imprint the question in your consciousness.

2. Perform the Noni Technique to Enhance Dreams and Sleep.

3. As you drift off to sleep, expect to have a dream that will address the question you wrote down.

4. When you wake up, whether in the morning or in the middle of the night, write down whatever dream you remember. At this point, do not try to edit your writing or figure out your dream—just write it down. If you remember nothing, write down how you feel. If you are not sensing any particular emotions, ask yourself what you *know* to be true. In your half-asleep state, don't worry that whatever you write down has anything to do with your question.

5. Sometime later that day, read what you wrote down. Look for a connection between the question you asked and the dream that you received.

# -65-

# Noni Eye Drops

Put Noni fruit juice in the eyes only if you dilute it with enough water and then allow it to rest. While resting, the pulp will settle to the bottom of the glass and the pulp-free Noni-water mixture can be used as Eye Drops.

## USE NONI EYE DROPS FOR:

Various conditions of the eye and particularly the surface of the eye including:
- Allergic reactions that affect the eyes.
- Conjunctivitis.
- Infections.
- Inflammation.
- Itchy eyes.
- Pinkeye.
- Tear gland infections.

## HOW TO MAKE AND
## APPLY NONI EYE DROPS:

1.  Pour a tablespoonful of Noni into a drinking glass.

2.  Measure four tablespoonfuls (one-quarter cup) of purified water in a measuring cup.

3.  Swirl the glass so that the Noni is moving in a circular direction. Meanwhile, pour the water into the Noni in a slow, steady, uninterrupted stream. Swirl a few seconds more to mix the liquids together.

4. Let the Noni-water mixture rest undisturbed for about five minutes while the pulp settles to the bottom of the glass. Use the pulp-free liquid at the top of the glass for Noni Eye Drops.

5. Use a clean eyedropper to collect some Noni Eye Drops from the top of the glass.

6. Place a few drops into the affected eye.

## MORE ABOUT NONI EYE DROPS:

Apply Noni Eye Drops several times a day if necessary. Keep the batch covered on the kitchen counter. After you have given the last application of Noni Eye Drops for the day, drink the Noni-water mixture that remains. Make a fresh batch of Noni Eye Drops each day you want to apply them.

As with other kinds of eye drops, Noni Eye Drops may sting for a few seconds. A soothing feeling should follow. Interestingly, some people don't feel the sting at all, or feel it only sometimes.

If you use bottled spring water kept at room temperature to make Noni Eye Drops, the temperature will be pleasantly cool on the eyes. Do not heat Eye Drops.

Noni Eye Drops consist of one tablespoonful of Noni and four tablespoonfuls of water mixed in a way that releases one of Noni's restorative energies. The mixture is called a 1:4 Dilution. Its restorative energy focuses Noni's beneficial compounds on the sense organs and nerves, which makes it ideal an application for the eyes.

Consider using the Noni Eye Poultice (page 269) in addition to Noni Eye Drops. Eye Drops are especially helpful for conditions on the surface of the eye, whereas the Eye Poultice can uplift the health of the entire eye.

For acute Eye Conditions, also follow the Procedure for Acute Conditions on page 75.

## AN ALTERNATIVE METHOD
## FOR APPLYING NONI EYE DROPS:

If you don't like taking eye drops or if you do not have an eyedropper, you may be grateful to know there is an alternative. This method is preferred for giving Noni Eye Drops to children. It may also be easier to use this method to administer eye drops to yourself.

1.  Prepare Noni Eye Drops following Steps 1, 2, 3 and 4 as described earlier in this chapter.

2.  Dip the edge of a cotton ball into the Noni-water liquid at the top of the glass. Wet only half the cotton ball. Use two cotton balls if you want to apply the Eye Drops to both eyes. Hold the cotton ball briefly over the glass to let any excess liquid drip off.

3.  Lie down on your back and place the wet side of the cotton ball on the corner of your eye beside the bridge of your nose.

4.  Gently press the cotton against your eye. This will release the Noni Eye Drops into your eyes in a gentle way that you can easily control. Meanwhile roll your eyeballs in circles to distribute the Noni Eye Drops around your eye.

5.  After your eyes have been bathed in Noni, the application is finished. However, if you have time, you could leave the cotton balls in place for about fifteen minutes to allow Noni's beneficial compounds to be absorbed into the area. When you are finished, remove the cotton balls and throw them in the trash.

# -66-
# The Noni Eye Poultice

A Noni Eye Poultice can be helpful for a variety of eye conditions as well as vision problems, for it raises the overall health of the eyes.

## USE A NONI EYE POULTICE FOR:

- Eyestrain.
- Glaucoma.
- Headaches behind the eyes.
- Macular degeneration.
- Pain in the eyes.
- Pinkeye and other eye and eyelid infections.
- Sties.
- Vision problems.
- Injuries, after first aid has been applied.
- Also, after eye surgery to promote recovery.

## HOW TO MAKE
## A NONI EYE POULTICE:

1.  Make a poultice pad about two inches wide, six inches long and four layers thick. You could unroll twenty-four inches of a two-inch-wide gauze bandage and fold it to fit these measurements. Alternatively, you could unfold a 4" x 4" gauze pad and refold it lengthwise into a 2" x 6" strip.

2.  Pour one tablespoonful of Noni fruit juice into a small glass. Measure one tablespoonful of purified water and

add this to the Noni. Swirl the glass briefly to mix the liquids together.

3. Let the Noni-water mixture sit for a few minutes to let some of the pulp settle to the bottom of the glass. The water gives volume to the mixture and helps separate out some of the pulp.

4. Carefully pour about half the Noni-water mixture into a bowl, leaving the bulk of the pulp behind in the glass.

5. Press the poultice pad into the bowl until it soaks up the Noni-water mixture. Then hold the pad over the bowl and gently squeeze out any excess liquid. The pad should be wet, but not soaking wet.

## HOW TO APPLY
## A NONI EYE POULTICE:

1. Bring the Eye Poultice and a dry napkin with you to the bed or couch. Lie down, close your eyes and place the poultice pad over your eyes.

2. Gently press the pad over your eyeballs and into the corners of your eyes to conform the pad to the contours of your face. Use the dry napkin to soak up any liquid that drips down your face.

3. Rest with the Eye Poultice in place for at least fifteen minutes. You could also apply the Eye Poultice just before going to sleep at night. If necessary, use a bandana to hold the pad in place. Or let the poultice fall off naturally during sleep, in which case put an old towel over your pillow so it doesn't get stained.

4. When the procedure is over, discard the Eye Poultice.

# MORE ABOUT THE
# NONI EYE POULTICE:

Some of the Noni-water mixture may seep into your eyes. This can enhance the therapeutic effect of the Noni Eye Poultice. To allow more Noni-water under your eyelids, gently press the Poultice into the inside corners of your eyes to release some of the liquid. Meanwhile, roll your eyes in circles. The Noni-water may sting, but it may not. Interestingly, you may feel the sting at some times and not others. Whether Noni will sting or not depends on the person, the type of eye condition and how the eyes may be feeling on that particular day.

For infections and serious conditions on the lid or the skin near the eye, you can use a Noni Compress (page 225), which consists of undiluted Noni. This would provide the area with a greater concentration of Noni beneficial compounds. However, if you use a Noni Compress on the eyes, do not press on the pad to release the undiluted Noni into your eyes. Noni pulp can irritate them. The Eye Poultice recipe separates out a bulk of the pulp. In addition, the pulp tends to stay trapped in the gauze material. Some Noni juice may remain on your face when you remove the Eye Poultice. This wipes off easily with a wet facecloth. The Noni Eye Poultice may help to relieve pain. If you are using it for this purpose put the leftover Noni-water mixture in the refrigerator. Use this cold mixture for a second application. The cool temperature of the Noni can enhance its analgesic effect. You can use the same poultice pad for a second application, but first rinse it out under running water to remove the spent Noni-water, as it may have absorbed toxins. The Noni Eye Poultice can be very soothing and relaxing. If used regularly, the Eye Poultice can raise the level of vitality in the eyes, thus preventing headaches due to eyestrain. A 2" x 6" poultice pad will fit most adults. Children will need a smaller size. If you are applying the Noni Eye Poultice to only one eye, use a poultice pad that is about 2" x 3" in size.

Drink the leftover pulpy Noni-water mixture just before applying the Eye Poultice. Count it as part of your daily serving of Noni. Drinking Noni enhances the beneficial effects of Noni applied topically.

# -67-

# The Noni Facial Formula

The Noni Facial Formula cleanses, removes dead skin cells (exfoliates), softens, moisturizes, and provides the skin with essential nutrients—all in a single time- and money-saving product.

## THE NONI FACIAL FORMULA CAN BE HELPFUL FOR:

- Acne and Pimples.
- Aging skin.
- Blotchy skin.
- Cleansing the skin.
- Dry skin.
- Rough skin.
- Wrinkled skin.

And as a daily facial cleansing program.

## HOW TO MAKE NONI FACIAL FORMULA:

1. Begin by turning a bottle of Noni upside down then right side up a few times to mix the pulp with the juice.

2. Use the end of a cotton swab to mix together:
   - One teaspoonful of Noni fruit juice.
   - One level teaspoonful of brown rice flour.
   - One-half teaspoonful of coconut oil (liquid at room temperature).
   - One-half teaspoonful of your favorite skin lotion.

# HOW TO APPLY NONI FACIAL FORMULA:

1.  Rinse your face with warm water.

2.  Apply about one-half teaspoonful of the Noni Facial Formula to your face. Gently massage the mixture all around your face in small circles. You can also apply it to your neck and upper chest.

3.  Use hot tap water to wet a facecloth, then wring it out and place it over your face. (This feels wonderful.)

4.  When the facecloth is no longer warm, rinse it in cold water. Use the cool washcloth to remove the Facial Formula from your skin. The cool temperature will help close and tighten your pores.

5.  Pat your face dry with a soft towel.

# MORE ABOUT THE NONI FACIAL FORMULA:

Noni fruit juice contains beneficial compounds specifically important for the skin. Brown rice flour is an excellent, all-natural, and inexpensive exfoliant. It contains essential amino acids; vitamins B1, B3 and B6; the minerals manganese, magnesium, selenium, phosphorus and iron; plus essential fatty acids.

Coconut oil, also called monoi oil, is a popular ingredient in many high-quality commercial skin preparations. For centuries, Polynesians have used coconut oil as a natural replacement for skin and hair oils. It quickly absorbs into the skin, and brings Noni's beneficial compounds along with it. Coconut oil solidifies at temperatures below 68° Fahrenheit (20°C) because it contains no emulsifiers to keep it in a liquid state. Therefore, you may need to soak the container in a bowl of hot water before measuring the amount of coconut oil you need. If you have Noni seed oil available, try adding a few drops to the formula.

The oil and lotion not only blend the Noni and brown rice flour together, but also lubricate the skin and allow the brown rice flour to cleanse the skin without irritating it. As dirt and dead skin cells are removed, Noni's beneficial compounds have better access to the skin cells. As a result of this procedure, your skin will feel soft, clean, moist and nourished.

Brown rice flour and coconut oil can be found in your local health food store.

Removing the Facial Formula with a cool facecloth will not only remove the leftover formula, but also leave behind a thin layer of coconut oil, which will help protect your skin and keep it soft and moist.

Noni Facial Formula can be kept in a cool dark place for a few days. Otherwise, keep it covered in the refrigerator. Double or triple the recipe in this chapter to make as much of the formula as you like.

This formula can be used to soften skin anywhere on your body. Your feet and legs may especially appreciate an application.

Try the Noni Facial with only one side of your face to discover the difference just one application can make.

# -68-
## The Noni Finger Soak

Use this procedure for one or more fingers.

### USE THE NONI FINGER SOAK FOR:

- Arthritis.
- Fungus.
- Infections.
- Injuries.
- Insect stings.
- Joint pain.
- Nail and cuticle conditions.
- Neuralgia.
- Stiffness.

### HOW TO MAKE AND APPLY
### THE NONI FINGER SOAK:

1. Start by placing a small pot of purified water on a hot stove.

2. Then find a bowl large enough to fit all your fingers. (If you bend your fingers and place your hand in the bowl, the top of your fingers should rest comfortably on the bottom of the bowl.)

3. Measure a tablespoonful of Noni fruit juice. Hold the affected finger over the bowl. Pour the Noni fruit juice

over the finger to coat it completely. Apply the noni to the entire finger, even if you have pain in only one part of it.

4.  Massage the Noni into the skin. (If your finger is injured or if massage is painful, omit this step.)

    With the thumb and forefinger of the other hand, squeeze the affected finger up and down, along its top and bottom, then its right and left sides. This method will increase circulation to the finger and enhance the absorption of Noni's beneficial compounds. Avoid massaging the painful area of the finger if touching it makes it feel worse. Periodically, re-coat the ailing finger with Noni by running the finger across the bottom of the bowl in order to pick up some of the Noni pulp that has fallen there.

    Spend a few minutes massaging each affected finger. (The Noni massage may feel so soothing you may want to massage all your fingers, whether or not they need it.)

5.  By now, the water on the stove should be hot. Remove your hand from the bowl and add enough hot water to the Noni in the bowl that the liquid will cover your fingers. The exact amount of water is not important. Test the temperature, and then replace your fingers in the Noni-water liquid. Continue to massage your fingers or let them rest in the bowl. If the water is too hot, cool down the Noni-water mixture by adding some cold water.

6.  After a few minutes, the Noni-water in the bowl will start to feel cool. If you'd like, add more hot water for a second Finger Soak.

# MORE ABOUT THE
# NONI FINGER SOAK:

Do not heat the water in a microwave. Test the hot liquid before putting a child's fingers into it.

After the Finger Soak is over, pour the Noni-water down the drain. Do not drink it. By now, most of Noni's beneficial compounds should have been absorbed into the skin and toxins from the fingers may have been released into the Noni.

Like other Noni applications, I have found that the Finger Soak can help reduce pain, promote healing, and increase joint flexibility.

The skin on your fingers may become temporarily wrinkled from being in the water. Your skin may also feel dry afterwards. If it does, apply a favorite moisturizer.

# -69-

# Noni First Aid
# for Minor Wounds

The information in this chapter should supplement—not replace—
the procedures you might read in a First Aid handbook.

When treating emergencies, even minor ones, it is essential
to use common sense and call upon the help of an Emergency
Medical Team if necessary.

## NONI CAN BE HELPFUL
## FOR MINOR WOUNDS, INCLUDING:

- Abrasions and scrapes.
- Bee stings.
- Bleeding.
- Blows and bruises.
- Burns.
- Cuts.
- Insect bites.

## HOW TO USE NONI FOR BLEEDING
## WOUNDS:

1. Apply basic first aid[26] to the bleeding wound:
   - If there is no foreign object in the wound, cover
     the wound with a clean, absorbent material and

---

[26] *American Red Cross: Community First Aid & Safety* (St. Louis: Mosby Lifeline, 1993), p. 148.

apply pressure. If no bones have been broken in the wounded area, raise the wound above the level of the heart to slow the blood flow. Try to calm the one who has been hurt. Assess how serious the wound is, what other injuries may be present, and if you need to call an Emergency Medical Team. If the bleeding doesn't stop, squeeze the nearby artery against the bone.

2. As soon as possible, pour Noni fruit juice over the wound. Also, make an impromptu Noni Compress by quickly pouring some Noni onto the cloth you are using to apply pressure over the wound.

3. Every ten seconds, remove the cloth, pour additional Noni over the wound, quickly replace the cloth and continue to apply pressure until the bleeding stops.

4. Give a Trauma Serving (page 95) to the injured person as soon as possible. Give Noni orally only if the individual is awake, able to drink and not in shock.

**Note:** Every time I use Noni for bleeding wounds, I am impressed by how quickly the bleeding stops. I have also found that the sooner Noni is applied to a wound, the faster the wound heals and the sooner pain seems to abate.

## HOW TO USE NONI FOR WOUNDS THAT HAVE STOPPED BLEEDING:

Noni fruit juice can stain wounded flesh a purplish color. The discoloration can remain for a while even after the wound has closed. To avoid this, try the following procedure:

1. Clean the wound with an antiseptic and cover it with an adhesive bandage to protect it.

2. Apply a Noni Compress over the adhesive bandage. The Compress should be big enough to cover the healthy skin adjacent to the wound. The body will transport Noni's beneficial compounds across body tissue to the wounded cells that need them. Leave the compress in place for about one-half hour.

## HOW TO USE NONI
## FOR BLOWS AND BRUISES:

Bruises involve internal bleeding. Apply a Noni Compress as soon as possible over the hurt area. Ideally, if you have Noni Paste available, apply it instead. The concentration of Noni beneficial compounds in Noni Paste can penetrate the body faster and more deeply.

1. Find a Noni Compress pad large enough to cover the wound. Use a gauze pad or fold a paper towel to the size you desire. In some cases, a cotton ball is just the right size.

2. Pour about one or two teaspoonfuls of Noni into a bowl (use more if necessary). Place the compress pad in the Noni and then cover the wound with the pulpy side of the pad next to the skin.

3. Secure the pad with first aid tape or a bandage.

4. Apply an ice pack over the wound to help with the pain. The cold can augment Noni's anti-inflammatory properties.[27] Give a Trauma Serving (page 95) as soon as possible.

---

[27] Neil Solomon, M.D. Ph.D., *The Pain Fighter: Find Natural Relief with Noni Juice* (Orem: Direct Source Publishing, 2005).

# HOW TO USE NONI FOR INSECT BITES:

Insect bites include mosquito bites, bee stings, wasp stings, spider bites and others.

1.  Wet a cotton ball (or half of one) with Noni and place it on the sting. If you have Noni Paste available, apply it instead.

2.  Secure the cotton in place with an adhesive strip or a piece of first aid tape.

If the sting is painful or if the victim is distressed or upset, offer a Trauma Serving (page 95). Meanwhile:

1.  Follow Step 1 above.

2.  When the cotton ball warms from body heat, soak another cotton ball in more Noni and apply. Do this as often as needed for pain. Additional applications provide more beneficial compounds to the area to replace those absorbed by the body. The cold temperature of a fresh cotton ball soaked in refrigerated Noni offers an additional analgesic effect.

3.  Finally, replace the cotton once again. This time, wet only half the cotton and place the wet side of the cotton on the bite. The dry portion of the cotton will absorb any excess Noni so it doesn't leak and stain clothing.

4.  Secure the cotton in place with an adhesive strip or a piece of first aid tape. Discard the used cotton balls.

# HOW TO USE NONI FOR MINOR BURNS:

For relatively minor burns, apply Noni generously to the area as described below. Severe burns should be treated by medical professionals. Offer Trauma Servings freely to saturate the body with Noni beneficial compounds.

If the burn is on a finger, pour enough Noni into a cup to submerge the burned finger in the Noni.

If the burn is elsewhere:

1. Soak an absorbent material in Noni fruit juice and place it over the burn. Use refrigerated Noni because it is cold, but Noni at room temperature is better than none at all.

2. When the material gets warm from body heat, leave the material in place and pour more Noni over it. (Replacing the material may irritate the burn.) Have paper towels handy to catch the Noni that will drip off.

3. Finally, when the pain has subsided, replace the material with a nonstick gauze pad soaked in Noni. Place another gauze pad or a paper towel over the pad to soak up any excess liquid. Secure this in place with first aid tape onto healthy skin. Otherwise, use another cloth or gauze bandage. If you need to transport a burn victim to the emergency room, keep the burn covered with a cloth soaked in Noni.

Some of the beneficial compounds in Noni fruit juice have proved to be very effective for helping the body heal quickly from burns, according to Dr. Ralph Heinicke, who has studied these compounds since the early 1970s.

In the case of burns, be generous with the amount of Noni fruit juice that you apply. Have extra paper towels handy to soak up any excess juice that drips off the body.

## MORE ABOUT USING NONI AS FIRST AID:

Remember to follow standard first aid procedures and call for help if necessary.

Drink a Noni Trauma Serving (page 95) as soon as possible after first aid has been applied. This will give your body a rich supply of beneficial compounds to aid the healing process. Be sure to do the Auto-dilution Procedure (page 133) with at least one sip of your Trauma Serving. This will direct Noni's beneficial compounds to the areas that need it most.

Noni is an excellent home remedy for first aid because of its ability to promote cell regeneration, reduce inflammation, fight infection and stop bleeding.

# -70-

# The Noni Foot Bath #1

If you cannot reach your feet, you will need someone to help you perform this procedure.

## USE THE NONI FOOT BATH #1 FOR A VARIETY OF FOOT CONDITIONS, INCLUDING:

- Arthritis.
- Athlete's foot.
- Blisters.
- Bone spurs.
- Bunions.
- Calluses.
- Cold feet.
- Dry skin.
- Gout.
- Poor circulation.
- Skin eruptions and infections.
- Sore feet.

## HOW TO APPLY NONI FOOT BATH #1:

First, an overview of this procedure: You will be inserting your foot in a plastic bag that contains Noni fruit juice. Then you will be placing your foot, with the bag, in a tub of hot water.

1.  Find a plastic bag suitable for this procedure. A one-gallon plastic resealable bag will fit most feet. Resealable bags are preferable to regular plastic bags because they tend to be stronger. If your feet are too large to fit in a one-gallon bag, you can use a small plastic garbage bag. You will need two bags if you are treating both feet.

2.  Pour one tablespoonful of Noni fruit juice in the plastic bag. Or use one ounce if your condition is painful or severe.

3.  Remove your shoes and socks and sit on the edge of the bathtub with your feet in the tub.

4.  Add about one-half inch of hot water to the tub. Rinse your feet in the water and then put each foot in a bag of Noni. The cold Noni will warm up very quickly in the hot water. Then wiggle your toes, flex your feet side to side and tap your feet on the bottom of the tub to distribute the Noni around your feet and to increase circulation to your feet. Do this often during the procedure.

5.  When the water starts to cool, add more hot water until the tub is once again very hot. Now the water level should be a little higher. Of course, do not make the water uncomfortably hot.

6.  Repeat Step 5 until the water level eventually reaches your ankles.

7.  When you are finished with the application, remove your feet from the plastic bags. Put your feet in the bath water to rinse off the Noni. Either dispose of the bags or rinse them out in case you want to reuse them for another Foot Bath.

8.  Dry your feet.

# MORE ABOUT THE NONI FOOT BATH #1:

Perform the Noni Foot Bath daily until your foot condition improves. Skin problems and acute foot conditions will likely improve more quickly than structural and chronic conditions. These conditions may require a daily Noni Foot Bath for a few weeks before significant improvement occurs.

Do not use the Noni Foot Bath if heat is contraindicated for your foot condition.

As the water level in the tub rises, the water pressure against the plastic bag will compress the bag against your foot. As a result, the Noni will be distributed all around your foot. However, if the plastic bag has a hole in it, the plastic won't cling to your foot as the water level rises. A hole will also enable water to seep into the bag. If only a few ounces of water get in, that's okay. You need not empty out the Noni and start over. Next time, use a stronger bag, or check the bag for leaks before you begin.

To help pass the time it takes to do this procedure, bring a book to read or something else to do while your feet are soaking.

When you are finished with the Noni Foot Bath, throw out the used Noni fruit juice. Do not drink it or apply it elsewhere on your body. The Noni may have absorbed toxins from your feet, and your feet should have absorbed most of the Noni beneficial compounds.

After the Noni Foot Bath, your feet will be red from the heat. You may notice that dry skin and calluses rub off more easily after soaking in Noni. Your feet may also feel more soft and smooth.

The water is added in stages to regulate the release of toxins from the foot, and to encourage these released toxins to move out through the bottom of the foot.

# -71-

## The Noni Foot Bath #2

This application works for a much longer period than Foot Bath #1.

### TRY THE NONI FOOT BATH #2 FOR:

- Arthritis.
- Athlete's foot.
- Blisters.
- Bone spurs.
- Bunions.
- Calluses.
- Dry skin.
- Fungus.
- Gout.
- Poor circulation.
- Skin eruptions and infections.
- Sore feet.

### HOW TO DO THE NONI FOOT BATH #2:

1. Before you go to bed for the night, pour a tablespoonful of Noni into a one-gallon plastic food storage bag. Resealable bags are stronger and preferable. Fill a second bag if you are going to do the procedure on both feet. You will also need an old towel and a pair of old, thick, comfortable socks.

2.  Lay the towel on the bed beneath the covers where your feet usually rest. The towel will prevent any Noni that may leak out from staining the linens. Get into bed.

3.  Insert one foot into a plastic bag. Put on a sock. The Noni will feel cold, but because it is cold, you will be able to feel where it is pooling. After putting on the sock, it usually pools around the heel. This is fine if your foot condition is located in your heel. Otherwise, spread the Noni around your foot by massaging it where you want it to go. You will feel its presence by its temperature.

4.  Repeat Step 3 with the other foot.

    **Optional:** Massage your feet for a few minutes each. This will help warm the Noni and distribute the Noni around your feet.

5.  In the morning, sit on the side of the bathtub, and with your feet in the tub, take off the socks and the plastic bags. Rinse your feet and dry them. Throw the plastic bags into the trash.

## MORE ABOUT THE NONI FOOT BATH #2:

Surprisingly, it does not take long to get accustomed to wearing plastic bags and socks on your feet all night long. This may be because the Noni feels so soothing on your feet. In addition to keeping the plastic bags in place, the socks will also help prevent the bags from breaking in case you have to get up and walk around after you have put them on.

You may find the Foot Bath #2 more convenient than Foot Bath #1 because you don't have to give it as much attention. In addition, your feet will be exposed to Noni for a much longer period, and your feet will soon warm up. On the other hand, the hot water used in the Foot Bath #1 helps Noni beneficial compounds to penetrate the body, and is very relaxing.

You could do Foot Bath #2 and put a heating pad between your feet. If you use a heating pad, you would only need to do the Foot Bath #2 for about half an hour. By then, the Noni beneficial compounds should be absorbed.

The instructions for this procedure suggest using one tablespoonful (one-half ounce) of Noni per foot, which should be sufficient for most conditions. For serious conditions, including pain, still try one tablespoonful first. If you then feel you need a more potent application, try one ounce of Noni per foot. Keep in mind that when using one tablespoonful of Noni, it is unlikely that any Noni will leak out of the plastic bags during the night. Leakage is more likely to occur with one ounce of liquid per bag.

You should notice some difference in the way your feet feel after only one application. Your skin and calluses will feel softer and your feet may feel more "alive" than ever before. Dry skin and calluses may be temporarily colored purple. If this bothers you, wash your feet with soap and water and rub them with a towel. You may find that dry skin and calluses peel off much more easily. Repeat the Noni Foot Bath #2 nightly for as long as it is needed.

Some people may find that their feet begin to itch while performing this procedure. Unless your skin is sensitive to plastic, the itchy feeling may indicate the release of toxins from your feet. Try massaging your feet for a few minutes, to help the toxins out. If the itchy feeling persists and becomes too uncomfortable, end the procedure. However, do try it again soon using less Noni (try a teaspoonful) because a release of toxins certainly indicates the technique is working.

# -72-
# The Noni Hand Treatment

Use this procedure for mild conditions or until you can make a recipe of Noni Paste and apply the Noni Procedure for Ailing Joints (page 241), which is preferred for more painful and serious hand conditions.

## TRY THE NONI HAND TREATMENT FOR VARIOUS CONDITONS OF THE HAND, INCLUDING:

- Arthritis.
- Fibromyalgia.
- Inflammation.
- Injuries.
- Neuralgia.
- Sprains.
- Tendonitis.

## HOW TO APPLY
## THE NONI HAND TREATMENT:

1. Turn a bottle of Noni upside down and right side up a few times to mix the pulp with the juice.

2. Measure one teaspoonful of Noni fruit juice and pour it into a one-gallon plastic food storage bag.

3. Insert your hand into the plastic bag. Gently press the plastic against your hand and massage the Noni to coat your entire hand.

4. To use your hand and fingers through the plastic, remove as much air from the bag as possible. Then gather the excess plastic that is around your wrist and twist the plastic into a few-inch long "rope," as you might twist closed a bag of chips. This will tighten the plastic around your wrist. Tuck the twisted plastic "rope" between the plastic bag and your wrist in order to secure the bag onto your hand.

5. Keep the Noni on your hand for at least fifteen to twenty minutes. Then dispose of the plastic bag and the spent Noni, and rinse your hand.

## MORE ABOUT
## THE NONI HAND TREATMENT:

Twisting and tucking in the open end of the plastic bag is preferable to using tape because you hand may get hot and start to sweat after a few minutes and you may need to open the bag to let in some air. The sweating, however, is an important part of this procedure as it helps the cells to release toxins.

One teaspoonful of Noni is enough to coat the hand without pooling in one area of the bag. Therefore, leaks should be minimal, but keep a napkin or paper towel handy just in case.

It is possible to perform the Noni Hand Treatment on both hands at the same time. Prepare two plastic bags, each with a teaspoonful of Noni. Before you insert your hands into the bags, have the television on or something ready to read to pass the time. It may be challenging to use your hands while both of them are incapacitated.

# -73-
# The Noni
# Headache Compress

Headaches are caused by many factors. It has been my experience that Noni is more helpful for some kinds of headaches than for others. Try this application to find out if the Noni Headache Compress will work for you.

## THE NONI HEADACHE COMPRESS MAY BE ESPECIALLY HELPFUL FOR HEADACHES:

- In the front of the head.
- Focused in the temples.
- Resulting from eyestrain.

## HOW TO MAKE AND APPLY THE NONI HEADACHE COMPRESS:

1. Make a compress pad about two inches wide and long enough to reach across your forehead to cover your temples. Try cutting a paper towel in half and then folding it to size, or use a gauze bandage or an old cotton T-shirt.

2. Turn a Noni bottle upside down and right side up a few times to mix the pulp with the watery portion of the juice. Pour a tablespoonful of Noni fruit juice into a bowl. Hold the compress pad by the ends and press the middle into the Noni in the bowl until the pad soaks up all the juice. Use the pulpy side of the pad to wipe up any Noni pulp that remains in the bowl.

3.  Put the compress pad back in the bowl and bring it with you to a comfortable place where you can lie down. Put your head on a towel to catch any Noni fruit juice that might drip out of the Headache Compress.

4.  Center the pad over your forehead and lay the ends of the pad over your temples. The pulpy side of the pad should be next to your skin. The Compress will soon warm with body heat, though its initial cool temperature can help relieve pain.

5.  Keep the Headache Compress in place for at least fifteen minutes or until the compress pad dries.

**Enhancing the Noni Headache Compress – Method #1:**
If you find the cool temperature of the Headache Compress helpful to relieve pain, try the following method, which adds the analgesic effects of cold temperature to the analgesic effects of Noni. You may need to cover yourself with a blanket during the treatment, as the cold compresses can make you feel cold all over.

1.  Prepare a second compress pad as described in Steps 1 and 2 above.

2.  Put some ice in a bowl and lay plastic wrap on the ice. Place both Headache Compresses on the plastic. This will keep them cold. Bring the bowl with you when you go lie down.

3.  Apply one Headache Compress. When it warms from body heat, replace it with the Headache Compress that is in the bowl of ice.

4.  Repeat Step 3 until you are finished with the procedure.

**Enhancing the Noni Headache Compress – Method #2:**
Use this method alone or with the Headache Compress. You could even use it along with Method #1.

1. Pour one teaspoonful of Noni into a bowl.

2. Tear a cotton ball in half and place it in the bowl to soak up all the Noni. Use the pulpy side of the cotton ball to wipe up the pulp that remains at the bottom of the bowl.

3. Put the cotton ball back in the bowl and bring it with you to the bed where your Headache Compress is waiting.

4. Place the Headache Compress on your forehead. Then place the Noni-soaked cotton ball on the top center of your head. Press the cotton ball against your head to help it adhere there. If you rest your head on a pillow, with your head slightly tipped up, then the Headache Compress and the cotton ball will likely stay in place without having to hold them.

   The top center of the head is an important energy point on the body. Placing Noni there can act as a way to help the head release any unwanted buildup of energy. Energy buildup in the head causes pressure that can manifest as headaches. Severe buildup can lead to vision problems, dizziness, hearing impairment, mental illness, imbalanced brain function and even cancer.

# MORE ABOUT THE NONI
# HEADACHE COMPRESS:

If Noni leaks out of the Compress, try massaging it into your scalp. This may also help your headache. When you are finished with the procedure, wipe any Noni pulp that remains on your forehead with a damp cloth and dispose of the compress pads.

If you are on the go and don't have time to do a Headache Compress, try rubbing a few drops of Noni seed oil on your temples, forehead, and sinuses. Noni seed oil can be obtained from most suppliers of Noni fruit juice.

In addition to the Headache Compress, consider taking a Trauma Serving (page 95). Also try the Noni Eye Poultice, to help ease eye pressure and light sensitivity due to the headache. You can do both the Eye Poultice and Headache Compress at the same time.

If your headache stems from a neck spasm, try a Noni Poultice (page 229) over the neck and cover it with hot towels. Or have someone give you a Noni Massage (page 309) on your neck and shoulders. In addition, try the Noni-clay technique for headaches (page 256). If your headaches are chronic, consider using the Procedure for Chronic Conditions on page 79. If your headaches are due to a buildup of toxins (including environmental pollutants), try Enhancing Noni's Effects with Water (page 141) or Hydrating with Noni (page 145) to help your body flush them naturally.

# -74-

# Noni Hemorrhoid Applications

## TRY THESE APPLICATIONS FOR:

- Hemorrhoids.
- Burning, itching and irritated anal tissue.

## HOW TO USE THE NONI HEMORRHOID APPLICATION METHOD #1:

1. Before bedtime, pour one teaspoonful of Noni fruit juice into a small bowl or medicine cup.

2. Press a cotton ball into the Noni until it soaks up all the Noni. Take the bowl with you to the bedroom.

3. Spread an old towel on the mid-portion of your bed's fitted sheet to protect it from being stained by the Noni.

4. Get into bed and lie down on your side.

5. Position the Noni-soaked cotton on the affected area. The pulpy side of the cotton ball should be against your skin. Press the cotton ball into your body or against it, as needed.

6. Keep the cotton ball in place while you sleep.

## HOW TO USE THE NONI HEMORRHOID APPLICATION METHOD #2:

1. Pour about one tablespoonful of Noni into a small bowl or medicine cup and put it beside the bathroom sink. Each time you are finished visiting the bathroom, do the following steps:

2. Dip a clean cotton ball into the Noni.

3. Sit on the toilet. Wipe the affected area with the cotton ball, or press the cotton ball against the affected area for several seconds.

## HOW TO USE THE NONI HEMORRHOID APPLICATION METHOD #3:

1. Pour one teaspoonful of Noni fruit juice into a small bowl or medicine cup.

2. Press a cotton ball into the Noni until it soaks up all the Noni. Take the bowl with you into the bathroom.

3. Place a sanitary napkin in your underwear.

4. Sit on the toilet. Position the Noni-soaked cotton on the affected area. The pulpy side of the cotton ball should be against your skin. Press the cotton ball into your body or against it, as needed.

5. Stand up carefully so the cotton ball stays in place. It is best to use underwear that fits snugly, so in case the cotton ball falls off your body it will stay trapped in

your underwear. The sanitary napkin will protect your clothing from any Noni that may leak out. Go about your day, enjoying the relief that Noni can provide.

## MORE ABOUT THE NONI HEMORRHOID APPLICATIONS:

You may expect some relief on the first application. However, constant contact between Noni and the affected area may be required to achieve and maintain comfort. This may mean repeating these methods often.

Men may object to the sanitary napkin suggested in Method #3. They may be able to omit that step if they put less Noni in the cotton ball. Then the Noni will be less likely to drip. Or simply use one of the other methods.

A cotton ball made of pure cotton is preferable to "cosmetic puffs," which look like cotton balls but are made of synthetic fiber. Cotton holds more Noni than synthetic fiber. It also tends to adhere better to the skin.

Soaking the cotton ball in refrigerated Noni fruit juice makes the cotton ball like a miniature cold pack, which has its own pain-relieving properties.

# -75-

# Noni for the Immune System

## USE NONI FOR THE IMMUNE SYSTEM:

- For fever.
- To help the body recover from illness.
- To boost the immune system.
- When an infant is distressed by teething.
- For pain throughout the body.
- For skin disorders that affect most, or a large portion of the body.
- For disorders affecting the entire body or a large portion of it, including conditions of the blood and lymphatic system.

## HOW TO MAKE THE NONI-LOTION MIXTURE FOR THIS PROCEDURE:

1. Turn a bottle of Noni upside down then right side up a few times to mix the Noni pulp throughout the juice.

2. Measure one ounce of Noni and pour it into a small bowl.

3. Measure one teaspoonful of body lotion.

4. Use a cotton swab to mix the lotion and Noni juice together. Mix well. You have now made Noni for the Immune System, which will be only slightly thicker than Noni juice alone.

# HOW TO APPLY
# NONI FOR THE IMMUNE SYSTEM:

1.  Bring the Noni-lotion mixture to the bathroom.

2.  It is best to shower and towel-dry first before doing this treatment so that the pores of your skin are clean, open and better able to absorb Noni beneficial compounds.

3.  Stand on an old towel to catch any Noni-lotion that drips. Use a teaspoon to scoop up a portion of the Noni mixture onto the palm of your hand. Spread the mixture one section of your body at a time. Cover your legs, buttocks, abdomen, chest, arms, neck, face and shoulders, and as much of your back that you can reach. (Or have someone apply it there for you.) Use both hands to rub the Noni-lotion mixture into your skin. Your skin will be wet with Noni-lotion.

4.  Apply extra Noni-lotion to the lymph glands on your neck, under your armpits and in your groin. Also apply some over your kidneys, which are located on your back on either side of the spine, just below your ribcage. The kidneys are an important organ of elimination that could use the support of Noni beneficial compounds during an illness. Most people should be able to reach their kidneys and apply the lotion there themselves.

5.  After you have covered all the sections of your body, apply additional coats until you have used all of the Noni mixture.

6.  Let your skin air-dry if possible (perhaps use this time to brush your teeth). Or don a bathrobe until the Noni-lotion soaks in. If necessary, use a small towel to wipe off any Noni pulp and Noni-lotion mixture that remains on your skin. Do not rinse yourself with water.

## MORE ABOUT
## NONI FOR THE IMMUNE SYSTEM:

After you do this procedure once, you will have a better idea how much Noni-lotion you need. You shouldn't have any Noni-lotion left over, but you may need to make more next time.

After you have spread the Noni-lotion over one section of your body, move to the next section of your body. Meanwhile, the skin on previously treated areas will absorb the Noni-lotion mixture by itself. If you find pieces of Noni pulp on your skin, rub them in. The lotion in the mixture will help the pulp disperse and soak in.

This application is ideal for babies and young children. Apply the Noni-lotion with massage and they may really enjoy it. Massage can stimulate the immune system as it promotes good circulation, moves lymph, and releases toxins.

However, releasing toxins is not the primary goal of this procedure. For adults, apply massage only until the lotion is spread around the skin, so as to discourage the release of toxins. Then the body can focus on stimulating the immune system.

Blanketing the body with an ounce of Noni fruit juice floods the skin with Noni beneficial compounds. This method activates and strengthens each individual cell. It also awakens the protective mechanism that surrounds the body as a whole. This procedure also activates the lymph glands as extra lotion is placed over them. The lymph glands are principle components of the immune system.

Your skin may be a bit sticky after this procedure, even after the Noni-lotion dries.  If you are ill and spending most of your time in bed or at rest, this shouldn't bother you.  If it does, wait about an hour, then wipe your skin with a damp cloth and then towel-dry.

# -76-

## Noni Massage

A Noni massage is a real treat!

### TRY A NONI MASSAGE FOR:

- Sore muscles.
- Low vitality.
- Illness.
- Nerve and muscle pain.
- When the body seems to radiate stress.

### HOW TO MAKE
### NONI MASSAGE OIL:

1. Measure one ounce of Noni fruit juice and pour it into a small drinking glass, bowl or plastic bottle.

2. Measure an ounce of your favorite unscented massage oil and pour it into the Noni. (Sesame oil or another lightweight oil is particularly nice.)

3. Mix the oil and juice together with your finger. Or, if you have added the oil and juice to a bottle, shake the bottle. Shaking will produce the best emulsion.

4. Pour Noni Massage Oil onto one section of the body at a time (for example the back of one leg, one arm or the shoulders). Smooth it over the skin quickly at first, so it

does not drip off. Massage that area completely before moving to the next (see Step 5). Make sure you are using plenty of Noni-oil mixture, so the skin feels wet.

5. You should notice the scent of Noni at first. After a few minutes, this scent will diminish as the body absorbs Noni's beneficial compounds. At this point, rub the area with a dry towel. This will remove any Noni pulp and excess Noni-oil from the skin, stimulate the skin and leave the skin feeling soft and smooth.

6. Then massage another section of the body, per Steps 4 and 5.

**Optional:** If the skin feels sticky after the massage is over, wipe the body, one section at a time, with a warm, damp cloth and towel dry once again.

## MORE ABOUT NONI MASSAGE:

The Noni-oil combination separates quickly. Remix it each time before you apply more to the body. However, don't worry that you cannot make a perfect emulsion. The two liquids will combine as you massage them into the skin.

In order for your body to obtain as many beneficial compounds as possible, a Noni massage should consist of about equal amounts of Noni and oil. This recipe suggests one ounce of each, which should be plenty for one whole-body massage for an adult. However, too much Noni in the mixture can make the Noni-oil combination too pulpy and sticky. Add a little more oil to the mixture if you think you should.

If you have Noni-oil left over and plan to use it within a few days, leave it at room temperature. Otherwise, store it in the refrigerator.

Expect muscle tension and stress to be relieved more quickly when incorporating Noni fruit juice into a massage. Noni also seems to cancel out the negative energies that seem to radiate from overly stressed muscles. In addition, Noni Massage Oil has a therapeutic effect on skin conditions and makes the skin feel wonderfully soft. Expect the muscles to release toxins, not only due to the massage itself, but also from the action of Noni's beneficial compounds. Drink extra water afterwards to help these toxins flush through the kidneys.

A massage therapist's hands will appreciate Noni Massage Oil because they won't tire as quickly and will benefit from the therapeutic effects of Noni.

Offer the person who will receive the massage an ounce of Noni to drink before the massage begins. This will enhance the benefits of Noni Massage. Drinking Noni enhances the beneficial effects of Noni applied topically.

# -77-

## The Noni Mini-Compress

This is a convenient way to use Noni on small areas.

### USE A MINI-COMPRESS FOR:

- Acne and pimples.
- Bee stings.
- Bruises, small.
- Boils and abscesses.
- Infected pierced-earring holes.
- Insect and spider bites.
- Irritated or infected moles.
- Puncture wounds.
- Ringworm.
- Small scars.
- Warts.

### HOW TO MAKE AND APPLY A NONI MINI-COMPRESS:

1. Use a half or a whole cotton ball, depending on the size of the affected area. (Use a whole cotton ball and use more Noni if the area is painful, so the area has access to a greater number of beneficial compounds.)

2. Pour about one-half teaspoonful of Noni into a medicine cup. Dip the cotton in the Noni so half of it is wet.

3. Place the wet side of the cotton over the target area and press it against your body to flatten the cotton. The dry portion of the cotton ball will soak up excess Noni to prevent the Mini-compress from leaking.

4. The surface tension of the wet cotton may be enough to keep it attached to your skin if you move around slowly. If the target area is underneath clothing or if you are active, secure the cotton with first-aid tape or with an adhesive bandage.

## MORE ABOUT THE NONI MINI-COMPRESS:

Most conditions for which this Mini-compress is applied clear up more quickly if you use the pulpier part of the Noni fruit juice. Noni pulp settles to the bottom of the bottle, so be sure to gently shake the Noni bottle before pouring Noni to apply to small areas.

Some moles, warts and small scars may require daily application for a few weeks before you notice significant changes. Try applying the Noni Mini-compress on these areas every night before bed, or try using Noni Paste (page 317). Acute problems may require only a few applications.

If you want to use the Mini-compress as first aid for an insect bite or small wound, simply tear off a piece of napkin or paper towel, quickly dip it in some Noni and apply it to the area in need. Then prepare a cotton ball as described above. Cotton holds more Noni over a smaller area than a paper towel can, and so is preferred.

You may have a few drops of Noni left over after Step 2. If so, you could use it following the Easy Skin Conditioner technique on page 259 or use it to make Quick Noni Paste (page 323).

If you would like to warm the Mini-compress, see Ways to Warm Noni (page 405).

# -78-

## The Noni Nail Treatment

Try this procedure on a single nail, all the fingernails, or the toenails.

### USE THE NONI
### NAIL TREATMENT FOR:

- Brittle and broken nails.
- Infected hangnails.
- Ingrown toenails.
- Nail fungus.
- Nail infections.
- Unhealthy cuticles.
- Unhealthy nails.

### HOW TO APPLY
### THE NONI NAIL TREATMENT:

1. Pour one or two teaspoonfuls of Noni into a bowl.

2. Tear cotton balls into pieces large enough to cover each of the nails you want to treat.

3. Dip one side of a cotton piece into the Noni fruit juice. It should be only half-wet. The dry part will soak up the excess juice, so it won't drip.

4. Place the wet side of the cotton on the nail to cover it. Press the cotton gently to adhere it to your nail.

5. Repeat Steps 3 and 4 for the other nails.

   **Optional:** Use the thumb and forefinger of your other hand to gently and repeatedly squeeze the sides of each nail. This will improve circulation to the nail and encourage the nail to absorb Noni's beneficial compounds, which will improve the benefits of the Noni Nail Treatment.

## MORE ABOUT THE NONI NAIL TREATMENT:

Keep the Noni Nail Treatment in place for at least fifteen to thirty minutes. It's a good procedure to do while you're reading or watching television.

For general nail care, do the Nail Treatment once every week or two, or every time you cut your nails. If you apply the Nail Treatment often, your nails should grow stronger and healthier.

If a nail problem is serious or painful, do the Noni Nail Treatment daily. Meanwhile, prepare a batch of Noni Paste (page 317) and then do Noni Cuticle Care (page 257), which is a more powerful application.

If you have just used nail polish remover, wash your hands well with soap before applying the Nail Treatment so that the chemicals in the nail polish remover do not interfere with Noni's beneficial compounds.

If you do this procedure while you are resting, the surface tension of the wet cotton may be enough to keep the cotton pieces in place. If you want to move around, secure the cotton to your nail with first-aid paper tape.

# -79-
## Noni Paste

Noni Paste provides a high concentration of Noni beneficial compounds in a form that is easy to apply topically. With so many uses for Noni Paste, it is a good idea to always have some on hand in the refrigerator.

### TRY NONI PASTE FOR:

- Acne.
- Athletic injuries.
- Blisters.
- Boils.
- Bruises.
- Burns.
- Canker sores.
- Carpal Tunnel Syndrome.
- Cuts and wounds (small).
- Foot fungus.
- Gum conditions.
- Herpes.
- Joint pain.
- Sore nail cuticles.
- Sore throat.
- Wrist pain.
- Mosquito bites.
- Pain in relatively small areas.

The above list comprises but a few of the many applications of Noni Paste. May these ideas inspire your imagination to try the Paste for other conditions.

# HOW TO MAKE NONI PASTE:

Before you begin, turn the bottle of Noni fruit juice upside down then right side up a few times. This will mix the pulp, which tends to settle to the bottom of the bottle, with the watery portion of the juice.

1. Pour one ounce of Noni fruit juice onto a dinner plate and spread it around by tilting the plate in different directions.

   Make sure the dinner plate has a deep enough indentation in the center that the liquid won't spill off. Don't use paper plates as the paper will absorb the liquid part of the juice, including its beneficial compounds.

2. Let the plate sit uncovered and outside the refrigerator for about a day. This will allow most of the water in the Noni juice to evaporate.

3. You will know when enough water has evaporated when you tip the plate and the Noni stays in place. Noni Paste should have the consistency of apple butter.

4. Use a rubber spatula to scrape the Noni Paste off the plate and into a small container. Cover the container with the plastic wrap touching the Noni Paste and store it in the refrigerator. Noni Paste can be stored this way for several weeks and used as needed.

This recipe makes about one to one and a half teaspoonfuls of Noni Paste, depending on how dry you let it become. Make extra batches as needed.

## MORE ABOUT MAKING NONI PASTE:

It is important to monitor the Noni fruit juice while it is becoming Noni Paste. If you let too much water evaporate from the Noni, it will dry out. This reduces the concentration and effectiveness of Noni's beneficial compounds. It is best start over again with fresh Noni fruit juice. Cover the plate with plastic overnight or if you have to leave the house for a while, and put the plate in the refrigerator. This will stop the evaporation. Remove the plate from the refrigerator and uncover it when you are ready to resume making Noni Paste.

How fast Noni fruit juice will become Noni Paste depends on air temperature and humidity. In hot, dry climates, it may take half a day. In normal humidity, it may take an entire day or longer. If you live in a very humid climate, you may be unable to make Noni Paste indoors. An alternative is to place the Noni fruit juice in sunlight. Doing so can vitalize the Noni Paste with the sun's energy. However, sunlight can evaporate water quickly, so be sure to keep a close eye on the forming Paste. It would also be wise to cover the bowl of Noni with a wire screen, or something similar that would keep out insects but still allow evaporation to occur. In the winter, evaporation tends to go much slower and can take up to three days. However, since you will not be ingesting Noni Paste, you can leave it out longer than you might if you were eventually going to drink it.

Do not try to evaporate the water from Noni using the stove. The temperature at which the water in the Noni fruit juice would steam away is high enough to destroy its beneficial compounds.

# HOW TO USE NONI PASTE:

1. Apply enough Noni Paste to cover the affected area.

2. Cover the Paste with an adhesive bandage if the area is small, or with a gauze pad or plastic wrap if the area is relatively large. Avoid letting the Paste dry out because then it becomes difficult to remove.

3. Keep the Paste in place for at least half an hour.

## MORE ABOUT USING NONI PASTE:

Noni Paste has many applications and is especially helpful for pain in localized areas.

Noni Paste has advantages over Noni Compresses and Noni Poultices. The Paste is easier to apply and less messy because it won't drip like the juice will. You can apply a thick coat of Noni Paste over an area, thus giving that area more Noni beneficial compounds per square inch than is possible with Noni Compresses. This makes Noni Paste especially helpful for small areas.

On the other hand, the advantages of Noni Compresses or Poultices include: they can be applied immediately (you don't have to wait a day to make Noni Paste), and they distribute Noni's beneficial compounds more evenly over a larger area.

Noni Paste is not recommended for rashes and broken skin. The concentrated Noni pulp in Noni Paste may irritate rashes, adhere to broken skin, and be more difficult to wash off. It would also be more likely to stain the skin purple.

When you are finished with the Noni Paste application, if the Paste is still moist, remove it with a damp cloth. Wipe the area a second and third time to remove any residue that might leave your skin feeling sticky. If the Paste is dry, remove it under running tap water or in the shower.

## MORE IDEAS FOR
## USING NONI PASTE:

- For painful areas, apply a thick layer of Noni Paste over the pain. Cover with gauze and first aid tape.
- For insect bites, apply a thick layer over the bite. Cover with an adhesive strip.
- For gum conditions, tear off a piece of a cotton ball that is large enough to cover the area you want to treat. Spread Noni Paste over one side of the cotton. Place the cotton inside your mouth with the Noni Paste against the affected gums.
- For a sore throat, spread Noni Paste on each side of the neck over points of pain as well as on swollen glands. Some people will enjoy the cool feeling of the Noni Paste over their sore throat. Other may find it soothing to cover the paste with a hot, moist towel.
- For foot fungus, cover the affected area with Noni Paste. Slip your foot into a plastic food storage bag. Put on a sock. Leave the Paste in place for at least an hour or overnight. (See also the Noni Foot Bath #2 on page 291).
- Noni Paste is also used for Noni Cuticle Care (page 257) and A Noni Procedure for Ailing Joints (page 241).

# -80-

## Quick Noni Paste

This paste recipe takes less time to make than regular Noni Paste does, though it is less concentrated.

### TRY QUICK NONI PASTE
### FOR CONDITIONS SUCH AS:

- Blisters.
- Boils.
- Insect bites
- Painful joints.

- Poison ivy.
- Rashes.
- Sprains.
- Wounds.

### HOW TO MAKE AND APPLY
### QUICK NONI PASTE:

1. In a small bowl, add three level teaspoonfuls of cornstarch and two teaspoonfuls of Noni fruit juice.

2. Use your finger to mix and press the ingredients together. They will form a mass that is shiny and sticks together into a single glob.

3. Use a spoon to apply the amount you need to the target area. The Quick Paste will stick to the body and spread slowly to cover the area. It will also form its own "skin."

4. Cover the Quick Paste with plastic or allow it to air-dry. When it dries, it will start to fall off in large chunks. Brush these off gently over the sink. The leftover powder on your skin easily rinses off with water. If you cover the Quick Paste, it will stay moist and you will have to rinse it off when the procedure is finished (after about an hour).

## MORE ABOUT QUICK NONI PASTE:

If you are allergic to corn or corn products, you should not use Quick Noni Paste, as it is made with cornstarch. You could substitute arrowroot powder, though the mixture is not as easy to work with. Avoid using flour as a substitute because a Noni-flour mixture does not stick to the skin very well.

Adjust the amount of Quick Paste that you make by using a different measuring spoon. For example, use a half-teaspoon measuring spoon to make less or a tablespoon to make more. Just keep the ratio the same: three parts of cornstarch to two parts Noni fruit juice. This proportion makes a mixture that is not too dry or too wet, and is easy to apply.

Quick Noni Paste is less concentrated than Noni Paste is, but it is ideal for skin conditions, especially for children. Quick Paste is soothing and not painful to apply. It allows Noni's beneficial compounds to enter the body while at the same time drawing toxins out. Its action is gentle, and may be especially helpful to those who are sensitive to other procedures.

# -81-

# The Noni Rash Plaster

Use the Noni Rash Plaster specifically for skin conditions.

## TRY A RASH PLASTER FOR
## CONDITIONS INCLUDING:

- Burns.
- Chicken pox.
- Dermatitis.
- Diaper rash.
- Eczema.
- Hives.

- Liver spots.
- Pimples and acne.
- Poison ivy.
- Psoriasis.
- Skin eruptions.
- Stretch marks.

## HOW TO MAKE AND APPLY
## A NONI RASH PLASTER:

1. Select a plaster cloth that will cover the affected area. You may use cheesecloth, an unfolded sterile gauze pad, a piece of an old T-shirt or a paper towel. A plaster cloth should be thinner than a pad used for compresses or poultices, so no need to fold it.

2. Pour some Noni fruit juice into a bowl. The amount of Noni you will need depends on the size of the plaster cloth you are using. Start with one-half tablespoonful of Noni and add more if needed. If your plaster cloth is bigger than four inches square, pour the Noni onto a dinner plate. This will make it easier to distribute the Noni evenly throughout the plaster cloth.

3.  Press the plaster cloth into the Noni fruit juice. Do not turn the cloth over.

4.  Hold the cloth over the bowl and squeeze the cloth gently to allow excess Noni juice to drip off.

5.  Lay the plaster cloth over the affected area to cover it. The pulpy side of the cloth should be touching the skin. The plaster will feel cold at first, but will soon warm up with body heat.

6.  Press the plaster cloth onto the skin and mold it around the contours of the body. Use a dry napkin to wipe up any Noni juice that drips.

    The plaster cloth will be slightly adhesive; perhaps just enough that you won't need to secure it in place. If you do want to secure it, don't use plastic wrap. In this case, you want the area to breathe—the skin heals better that way. Try wrapping the plaster cloth with a gauze bandage instead. Apply additional plaster cloths as needed to cover all of the affected skin. The Noni Rash Plaster can cover a considerably large portion of the body if necessary.

7.  Leave the plaster cloth in place until it dries. Then rinse out the cloth (or, if using a paper towel, discard it), then soak the cloth in more Noni and reapply.

# MORE ABOUT THE
# NONI RASH PLASTER:

Apply the Noni Rash Plaster as often as needed.

For contagious rashes such as poison ivy, you may leave the Rash Plaster in place even when it dries out. This may prevent the rash from spreading. However, a wet plaster seems to work better to control itching.

Think twice before using the Noni Rash Plaster for pimples or acne on the face. Noni fruit juice can stain open skin a purple color.

For diaper rash, apply the Noni Rash Plaster on the reddened area. Then put on the diaper. The diaper will hold the Plaster in place. When you change the diaper, throw out the plaster cloth. Then reapply the Rash Plaster using a clean plaster cloth soaked in more Noni juice. My babies' diaper rashes have cleared up quickly using this technique.

To warm the Rash Plaster before placing it on your baby's bottom, prepare the Plaster as in Steps 1 through 3, but use a glass bowl. Add a few inches of very hot tap water to the bathroom sink. Place the bowl, which contains the Noni-soaked Rash Plaster, in the hot water to warm. Be sure none of the water gets into the bowl. In the meantime, clean up the baby. By the time you are ready to apply the Noni Rash Plaster, the plaster cloth should be warm. Test its temperature before you place it on the baby.

# -82-

# The Noni Scalp Application

Don't worry, this procedure will not turn your hair purple!

## TRY THE NONI SCALP APPLICATION FOR SCALP CONDITIONS, INCLUDING:

- Dandruff.
- Eczema.
- Itchy scalp.
- Psoriasis.
- Scalp sores.

## HOW TO PERFORM THE NONI SCALP APPLICATION:

1. Pour some Noni fruit juice in a medicine cup or small plastic cup. You will need at least one tablespoonful. Use as much as two ounces if your condition occurs throughout your scalp, if you have a lot of hair or if your condition is relatively severe.

2. Wrap a towel around your neck and shoulders.

3. Hold the cup with the Noni over your head. Part the hair over a section of your scalp. Pour some of the juice on this area so the Noni makes direct contact with your skin. As you pour the juice on, massage it into your hair so it does not drip off your head.

4. Repeat Step 3 with different sections of your scalp. Apply the Noni to your entire scalp, or just those areas that need it. Put a second and third coat of juice over problem areas.

5. When you have applied Noni to all the areas that need it, massage it into your scalp for a few minutes.

6. Brush or comb your hair. Then let it air dry, or cover your head with a towel or an old shower cap.

7. Keep the Noni on for at least fifteen minutes, overnight, or just until it dries. Then rinse out the Noni fruit juice and wash your hair.

## MORE ABOUT THE
## NONI SCALP APPLICATION:

Repeat this procedure daily until the condition improves.

You may need someone else's help to do this procedure, especially if you find it difficult to reach your arms up over your head.

If you have little or no hair, use the Noni Rash Plaster (page 325) instead.

Besides having a therapeutic effect on scalp conditions, the Noni Scalp Application may also help to alleviate headaches.

If you do this procedure before bed, cover your pillowcase with a towel to prevent the juice from staining it.

Noni fruit juice applied to your scalp acts somewhat like styling gel—with a fruity fragrance.

In researching whether Noni can be used safely on hair, I collected many hair samples that included natural, treated, as well as gray hair. Part of each sample was soaked in Noni fruit juice for over twenty-four hours, and then studied. I also examined the samples under a microscope. Noni appeared to have no negative effect on the natural and gray hair samples. I noticed that after using Noni on my own scalp (I kept it there until it dried, and then washed it off), my natural hair seemed softer and to have more "body."

The effects of Noni on treated hair varied and were inconclusive. This is not surprising, since there are so many different kinds of hair treatments. Just to be safe, those who have treated hair and wish to do the Noni Scalp Application should wash off the Noni after about twenty to thirty minutes. This is plenty of time to allow the Noni to work on your scalp, while not interfering with your hair treatment.

# -83-

## The Noni Sitz Bath

A bath of Noni fruit juice? Well, not exactly.

### TRY THE NONI SITZ BATH FOR:

- Childbirth recovery.
- Conditions of the anus.
- Conditions of the bladder and urethra.
- Conditions of the male genital organs.
- Conditions of the vagina and labia.
- Hemorrhoids.
- Hernias.
- Menstrual cramps.

### HOW TO TAKE A NONI SITZ BATH:

1. Fill the bathtub with three inches of hot water. Use water that is hotter than you would normally add to a bathtub.

2. Pour one to three ounces of Noni fruit juice into the bath water.

3. Step into the water. Sit down slowly to give yourself time to acclimate to the hot water. When you are seated, keep your knees bent so that the only parts of your body in the water are your feet and bottom.

4.  Rest in the tub for at least fifteen minutes or until the water cools. Every so often, move your hands through the water to keep the Noni pulp well mixed throughout the bath water. The Noni water will be very soothing to your bottom.

## MORE ABOUT THE NONI SITZ BATH:

If you think you may get chilly while sitting in a tub with relatively little water, wear an old t-shirt or wrap yourself with a towel that you don't mind getting wet.

You can also add other herbs or herbal teas to the bath water that are appropriate for your condition.

Bending your knees so that your feet are also in the water is therapeutic for two reasons. First, the feet have energy points and meridians that connect to every organ and area of the body. The heated Noni-water will indirectly stimulate the entire body through these points. Second, having your feet in the hot Noni-water will draw energy down your body. Energy often gets stuck in the head if we have an active mind, or if we tend to get caught in thoughts or other mental habits such as worry, impatience or being chronically upset. When energy is caught in the head, then the body has difficulty moving it to areas that need it to heal.

When our feet are stimulated, as they are in this application, this energy is given a pathway to move downward, away from the head. The body is then free to use this energy elsewhere. This technique directs that energy to your bottom—as that is the only other part of your body in the hot bath.

When the bath is over, you don't have to rinse yourself off before getting out. The Noni pulp will settle to the bottom of the bathtub and will not coat your body. The Noni-water that remains on your skin may also be mildly therapeutic.

# -84-

## The Noni Topical Splash

The Noni Topical Splash is helpful for skin conditions that cover relatively large areas or when you need quick relief for skin conditions when on the go.

### USE A NONI TOPICAL SPLASH FOR:

- Allergic reactions.
- Chicken pox.
- Dermatitis.
- Eczema.
- Pimples and acne.
- Poison ivy.
- Psoriasis.
- Rashes.
- Scalds.
- Skin irritations.
- Sunburn.

### HOW TO APPLY A
### NONI TOPICAL SPLASH:

1. Pour an ounce of Noni fruit juice into a small glass.

2. Measure three tablespoonfuls (one and a half ounces) of purified water and pour this into another glass.

3. Swirl the glass of Noni juice so it is moving in a circular motion. Meanwhile, pour the water into the Noni in a slow, steady, uninterrupted stream. Continue to swirl the glass for another few seconds to mix the liquids together. You have now made a 2:3 Dilution of Noni.

4. Let the Dilution rest for at least five minutes so the pulp can settle to the bottom of the glass. Then pour the pulp-free portion of the liquid into a glass tincture bottle with an eyedropper for a lid. You have now made Noni Topical Splash. Drink the pulpy portion that is left over as part of your daily serving of Noni.

5. Whenever you need to, use the eyedropper to place a few drops of Topical Splash on your skin. Then gently spread it over the affected area with your fingertips.

6. When the Topical Splash dries (usually about a minute later), apply it a second or third time if necessary.

## MORE ABOUT THE NONI TOPICAL SPLASH:

Carry the bottle of Topical Splash with you and use it as often as needed. Keep it refrigerated whenever possible.

Don't shake the Noni bottle before pouring the juice to make the Topical Splash. Skin conditions respond better to the watery part of the Noni fruit juice, found at the top of a bottle of Noni that has been left undisturbed. Using the pulpy part of the juice can leave pulp remnants on the skin. This is not a bad thing, but it can look unsightly. If you end up with pulp on the skin, brush it off when the Topical Splash dries.

Noni by itself can feel sticky when applied to the skin. Adding one and a half parts of water dilutes the Noni just enough to keep it effective without becoming sticky. Nor will this ratio of Noni and water give the skin a purple cast. On a more metaphysical level, this ratio of Noni and water, called a 2:3 Dilution, releases a restorative energy that focuses on the skin.

The Topical Splash can leave the skin feeling soft and smooth. It can also reduce itchiness and irritation on contact.

# -85-

# The Noni
# Tummy Treatment #1

Use this Noni Tummy Treatment on the lower abdomen (on and below the bellybutton).

## USE THE NONI
## TUMMY TREATMENT #1 WHEN:

- A child is ill.
- A child refuses to drink Noni.
- Drinking Noni causes nausea.
- You experience a cleansing reaction.
- You are unable to take liquids orally.
- You are hypersensitive to drinking Noni.
- You want to support the body through a fever.

**The Noni Tummy Treatment #1 is also helpful for:**

- Conditions of the intestine and abdomen.
- Endometriosis.
- Heavy metal or chemical toxicity.
- Systemic candidiasis.
- Intestinal parasite infestation.

# HOW TO APPLY THE
# NONI TUMMY TREATMENT #1:

1.  Select a compress pad:
    *   Use a 2" x 2" gauze pad for infants and a 4" x 4" gauze pad for babies.
    *   For children, teens and adults who have somewhat flat tummies, use one paper napkin. Paper napkins are about six inches square and large enough to cover the required area.
    *   Adults with larger tummies can use a paper towel.

2.  Heat a glass bowl by pouring boiling water into it.

3.  Turn a bottle of Noni upside down then right side up a few times to mix the pulp with the watery portion of the juice.

4.  The bowl should now be hot. Pour out the water and quickly dry the bowl.

5.  Pour about one tablespoonful of Noni fruit juice into the heated bowl. (Use less for children; use one ounce if you are using a paper towel.)

6.  Place the compress pad on the Noni fruit juice and gently press down on the pad to help it soak up the Noni.

7.  When you remove the pad from the bowl, wipe up any pulp that remains in the bowl with the pulpy side of the pad.

8.  Place the wet pad over the lower abdomen. The top inch of the pad should cover the bellybutton. (Overweight individuals should center the compress pad over the

bellybutton.)  The pulpy side of the pad should be touching the skin.

9.  Cover the compress pad with plastic wrap, and then with an old hand towel to keep it warm.

## MORE ABOUT THE
## NONI TUMMY TREATMENT #1:

You can prepare the Noni Tummy Treatment with undiluted Noni or with equal parts of Noni and water.  It is easier and preferable to use undiluted Noni when applying the Tummy Treatment on babies and children.  Adults who are using a paper towel may prefer to dilute the Noni with water for a more economical application.  See "How to Make a Noni Poultice" on page 229 for instructions for making a 1:1 Dilution.  Diluting the Noni will also help Noni's beneficial compounds be absorbed into the adult body.

Keep the Tummy Treatment in place for about half an hour. Apply it once or twice a day or as often as needed until the condition improves.

People who prefer to sleep on their back could apply the Tummy Treatment at night before going to bed.

If the compress pad cools off by the time you are ready to apply it, leave the pad in the bowl of Noni. Then place the bottom half of the bowl in a container or sink full of hot water. Apply the compress pad when it is warm enough.

For babies who are ill, give the Tummy Treatment each time you do a diaper change. A gauze pad can completely cover the baby's abdomen. The diaper will hold the Tummy Treatment in place, so you won't need plastic wrap for that purpose. (Besides, the plastic might irritate their delicate skin.  However, you could use a piece of plastic folded to the same size as the compress pad to cover the Tummy Treatment.) This will prevent the diaper from soaking up the Noni. The diaper will protect the clothing from being stained, but you may need a larger sized diaper than usual.

Noni Tummy Treatments are the next best thing to drinking Noni for two reasons. First, Noni's beneficial compounds enter the body through the bellybutton more quickly than through skin elsewhere on the body (except under the tongue). Second, the Noni beneficial compounds that enter the body through the bellybutton tend to remain in the abdominal area and work there, rather than spreading throughout the body as they do when taken orally. See also The Noni Tummy Treatment #2.

# -86-
## The Noni Tummy Treatment #2

So that's what bellybuttons are for!

## USE THE NONI TUMMY TREATMENT #2 FOR CONDITIONS OF THE ABDOMEN:

- Abdominal pain (be sure to also consult a medical professional).
- Bloating.
- Constipation.
- Diarrhea.
- Fever.
- Indigestion.
- Parasites.
- Yeast.

**Tummy Treatment #2 is preferred over Treatment #1 for:**

- Those who are overweight.
- Children who won't lie still long enough to keep a compress pad in place.

## HOW TO DO THE
## NONI TUMMY TREATMENT #2:

1.  Pour about one teaspoonful of Noni into a glass bowl.

2.  Select a cotton ball large enough to completely fill and cover the bellybutton. Use half a cotton ball for youngsters.

3.  Press the cotton ball into the Noni. The cotton ball should be saturated with Noni and may be dripping wet.

4.  Bring the bowl with the Noni and the cotton ball to a comfortable location where you can lie down for a while. Also bring a paper napkin or paper towel to wipe up any Noni that drips, and to clean up after the procedure is over.

5.  Lie on your back and insert the Noni-soaked cotton ball into your bellybutton.

If you must get up while wearing the Tummy Treatment #2, hold a paper napkin over your bellybutton.

## MORE ABOUT THE
## NONI TUMMY TREATMENT #2:

If the idea of applying cold Noni fruit juice to your bellybutton sounds uncomfortable, warm the Noni first. See Ways to Warm Noni for More Comfortable Topical Applications on page 405. Be sure to check the temperature of the Noni before you place it on a child's body—or your own, for that matter.

If you perform this application before taking a nap or going to bed at night, place an old towel beneath you to protect the bed linens from being stained in case the cotton ball falls out.

Keep the cotton ball in place for at least fifteen minutes, and longer if possible. For infants, a diaper can secure the cotton ball in place. Use first aid tape or an adhesive bandage on children if they are unwilling to lie still during the treatment.

The Noni Tummy Treatment #2 is easier to apply than Treatment #1, although #1 may be preferred because having a Noni Compress on your stomach can feel very soothing. In addition, some people may feel uncomfortable with the idea of putting a Noni-soaked cotton ball in their bellybuttons. On the other hand, the oddity can intrigue some children enough that they will allow you to do it.

# -SECTION 3-

# INTERNAL APPLICATIONS OF NONI

Drinking Noni and applying it topically are the two most obvious uses of Noni. However, this remarkable juice can also be therapeutic in ways that one might not expect. If it seems too odd to use Noni in some of the ways suggested in the following chapters, don't think of Noni as a juice. Think of it as a liquid that contains extraordinary beneficial compounds.

This section describes procedures for many internal applications of Noni fruit juice. The applications are listed alphabetically. When you try one of these methods, use it at least three times before judging how well you think it works.

When you use internal Noni applications, also plan to drink Noni using one of the procedures from Section 1 that best suits your condition. Oral and internal Noni applications will enhance each other's benefits. Internal applications also draw the beneficial compounds from the Noni that you drink to those parts of the body where the Noni is applied. So drink half a serving immediately before the internal application and the other half immediately afterwards.

# -87-

## The Noni Douche

Yes, Noni can help in this area as well.

### USE A NONI DOUCHE
### FOR CONDITIONS SUCH AS:

- Menstrual cramps.
- Vaginal itching.
- Vaginal odor.
- Yeast infections.
- Personal hygiene after sexual intercourse.

## HOW TO USE A NONI DOUCHE:

1. Fill a douche bag with warm, purified water. Add one or two ounces of Noni fruit juice to the bag. Attach the tube to the bag and attach the applicator to the tube.

2. Find a position in the shower or bathtub that is comfortable. You may stand, squat, kneel on one knee, or lie on your back—many positions will work. You can even douche over the toilet seat.

3. Hold the douche bag above your waistline. Hold the tube lower than this and allow any air in the tube to empty out. When the Noni-water mixture starts to come out, quickly insert the applicator into your body. Insert it as far as it will go comfortably.

4. Move the applicator as necessary to allow the liquid to cleanse the entire area. The Noni-water liquid will spill out of your body as you perform the douche.

## MORE ABOUT THE NONI DOUCHE:

Have a sanitary pad or panty liner ready to wear when you are finished. Any juice that leaks out could stain your clothing or the bathroom carpet.

Symptoms can be alleviated seconds after douching, although sometimes it takes a few hours to feel relief. For more stubborn or serious cases, try the Noni Vaginal Implant (page 389) or the Noni Tampon Implant (page 393).

For menstrual cramps and other symptoms of PMS, try the Procedure for Chronic Conditions (page 79). Use the Noni Douche daily, starting two weeks before you expect menstruation to begin.

The Noni Douche is not a contraceptive.

# -88-
## Noni Ear Drops

Noni Ear Drops are effective for children and adults as well as for pets. This chapter offers three methods for using Noni Ear Drops on yourself or others, with or without an eyedropper.

## TRY NONI EAR DROPS
## FOR CONDITIONS SUCH AS:

- Chronic dizzy spells.
- Ear infections.
- Ear pain.
- Earaches.
- Headaches.
- Impaired hearing.
- Loss of hearing.

## HOW TO APPLY NONI EAR DROPS:

**METHOD #1**
1.  Fill a clean glass eyedropper with Noni fruit juice.

2.  Hold the end of the eyedropper in a bowl of hot tap water to warm the juice.

3.  Put a drop of the warmed Noni on the back of your hand to test its temperature. If the Noni is still too cold, put the dropper back under the hot water. If the Noni feels too hot, wait a minute while the air cools it off, then retest.

4.  Have the person who is to receive the Noni Ear Drops lie down, facing sideways with their head on a pillow. Place a towel on the pillow, as any Noni that may leak out of the ear will stain the pillow or bed clothes.

5.  Apply the Noni Ear Drops:
    *   For children, place two or three drops of warm Noni fruit juice inside the ear.
    *   For adults, keep adding drops until the ear canal fills with juice.

6.  With your fingertip, gently rub behind the ear and just underneath it to work the juice towards the eardrum.

7.  Pack the ear with a small piece of cotton.

8.  Repeat Steps 5, 6 and 7 with the other ear.

## METHOD #2
Use this method if you don't have an eyedropper.

1.  Warm about two teaspoonfuls of Noni fruit juice as described in the information box below.

2.  Soak the end of a cotton swab in the warm Noni. Touch the wet end of the cotton swab against your cheek to check the Noni's temperature.

3.  If you are applying the Noni Ear Drops to yourself, lie on your side and drape a towel over your neck and behind your ear. Press the wet end of the cotton swab against the opening of your ear canal. This will cause some of the Noni to drip into your ear.

4.  You may have to dip the cotton swab back in the Noni juice and repeat this step a few times until your ear is filled. If you are using this method on someone else, simply hold the cotton swab over the ear canal's opening. Then squeeze the cotton tip to release the juice into the ear.

5.  Use the other end of the cotton swab to wipe up any Noni on the outer ear that didn't make it into the ear canal.

6.  With your fingertip, gently rub behind the ear and just underneath it to work the juice towards the eardrum.

7.  Pack the ear with a piece of cotton.

8.  Repeat this procedure for the other ear, using a new cotton swab.

---

### HOW TO WARM NONI EAR DROPS
### FOR METHODS #2 AND #3:

1.  Heat a glass bowl or teacup by filling it with boiling water or very hot tap water.
2.  After about fifteen seconds, pour out the water. The cup should be very hot.
3.  Quickly dry the cup and pour in one or two teaspoonfuls of Noni fruit juice.
4.  After a few seconds, the Noni will get warm. Use it before it cools.

---

**METHOD #3**
This method does not employ an eyedropper and is not recommended for children because of the small size of their ears.

1. Warm about two teaspoonfuls of Noni fruit juice as described in the information box on the previous page.

2. Tear apart a cotton ball to make two pieces the right size to plug the opening of each ear.

3. Dip one cotton piece into the warmed Noni fruit juice so that half of it is wet. Touch the wet cotton to your cheek to check its temperature.

4. Lie on your side and hold the wet cotton over your ear canal. The wet side of the cotton should be facing your body. Squeeze the juice into your ear.

5. Then pack the same piece of cotton gently inside your ear, with the wet side facing in.

6. With your fingertip, gently rub behind your ear and just underneath it to work the juice towards the eardrum.

7. Repeat Steps 3 through 6 with your other ear.

## MORE ABOUT NONI EAR DROPS:

Apply Noni Ear Drops two or three times a day as needed.
Before pouring Noni fruit juice for Noni Ear Drops, gently turn the Noni bottle upside-down and right-side-up a few times. A mix of the Noni juice and pulp makes the best Noni Ear Drops. Avoid shaking the Noni bottle so much that air bubbles form. The ear canal is a relatively small area. Air bubbles in the Ear Drops would prevent the Noni from reaching the entire ear.

Massage any unused Noni Ear Drops behind the ear as well as on the glands on the left and right sides of the neck. Or make Mini-compresses and put them on these areas.

My children have enjoyed relief from minor ear infections after only one or two applications. (This was verified by examining the ears with an otoscope.) Several applications may be necessary for more serious conditions.

Chronic ear conditions may require Noni Ear Drop applications daily for a few weeks. Meanwhile, follow the Procedure for Chronic Conditions (page 79). For acute ear conditions, also follow the Procedure for Acute Conditions (page 75).

If an ear condition is painful, apply Noni Ear Drops and then apply a Noni Compress (page 225). One way to do this is to use a thin compress pad that is about four inches square. Gently press the Noni-soaked compress pad around the ear so it conforms to the contours of the ear. Another option is to apply a small Noni-soaked cotton ball in the indentation behind the earlobe. For children, you could also dab a bit of Noni Paste behind the earlobe. Do this when they are asleep and put a towel underneath their head to protect the linens. In the morning, expect to wipe up any Noni Paste that spreads onto their hands and face if they move around during sleep.

Apply the Noni Ear Drops daily for a few days, even after the pain subsides.

If a physician examines your ears after you have put Noni Ear Drops in them, let the doctor know that you have used Noni. The ear canal may contain purple remnants of Noni pulp. Sometimes, however, there is no trace of Noni in the ear. The ear seems to have eagerly absorbed the Noni, pulp and all.

# -89-

## The Noni Enema

A relatively small amount of Noni fruit juice in an enema bag can make a big difference.

## TRY A NONI ENEMA FOR CONDITIONS SUCH AS:

- Constipation.
- Detoxification.
- Heavy metal poisoning.
- Inflammation.
- Parasites.

## HOW TO USE A NONI ENEMA:

1. Add warm water to a standard, two-quart enema bag until it is nearly full. If your tap water is chlorinated, use heated purified water. Test the temperature of the water in the bag with your finger to make sure the water isn't too hot.

2. Add one tablespoonful of Noni fruit juice to the enema bag.

3. Attach one end of the enema tube to the bag and the other end to the enema applicator. Lubricate the applicator with an herbal ointment. Don't use a mentholated ointment—it will sting!

4. Hold the enema bag over the sink and allow any air that may be trapped in the bag to exit through the tube. When Noni-water liquid starts to come out of the bag, squeeze the stopper that is attached to the tube. This will stop the flow of the liquid.

5. Hook the enema bag onto the shower door or the bathroom door handle. Place an old towel on the bathroom floor. Then find a comfortable position: Try lying on one side or on your back, or kneeling on your hands and knees.

6. Insert the applicator into your rectum. Release the stopper that is attached to the tube. Try to relax in order to allow the liquid to enter your intestines. Squeeze the stopper as needed to regulate the flow of the Noni-water liquid into your body.

7. When you feel an urge to expel the liquid, squeeze the stopper and remove the applicator from your body. Try to retain the liquid for a few minutes. If the urge passes, and if you were able to successfully retain the liquid, try massaging your lower abdomen. This will help break up accumulation in your intestines. Massage in the direction that food usually goes when passing through the intestines—looking down at your abdomen, this would be in a clockwise circle. Insert more Noni-water when you can.

8. When you are ready, expel the enema into the toilet. Some people are able to retain the entire contents of the enema bag. Others can only retain a portion of the enema at a time.

# MORE ABOUT THE NONI ENEMA:

Noni fruit juice added to an enema can help the intestines feel soothed and peaceful, despite the relative stress of the enema itself.

If your colon is very unhealthy, think twice about filling the enema bag a second time and doing an enema immediately following the first. It may be too much activity for the intestines at one time.

Experiment with different amounts of Noni in the enema bag. This way you can find an amount that suits you best.

You may add Noni along with other natural substances that are sometimes included in enemas, such as sea-salt and liquid chlorophyll.

You may find parasites expelled into the toilet bowl, but microscopic parasites may also be eliminated (which you obviously won't be able to see).

Here is one suggestion for how often to use a Noni Enema:

1. Use the enema once a day for a week.

2. Then take the enema every other day for a couple of weeks.

3. Gradually decrease the frequency of the enemas to once a week.

4. If symptoms recur, repeat this schedule.

Or, try a series of enemas and gradually increase the amount of Noni you add with each application. Start with a tablespoonful and increase the amount by one tablespoonful increments until you are using as much as eight ounces of Noni per enema bag. Then finish the series by decreasing the amount by one tablespoonful each time. Adjust these amounts to meet your personal needs.

During a detoxification crisis, Noni enemas can help calm and stabilize the body. In this case, start with two ounces of Noni fruit juice in the enema bag. The second day, use one ounce and the third day, add only one tablespoonful. Decreasing the amount of Noni used in a series of enemas helps to slow down a cleansing reaction.

Noni fruit juice may also be used for colonic irrigation, which is a special procedure performed by a Colon Therapist. A Noni Colonic Irrigation is more thorough and effective than a Noni Enema, and reaches farther up into the intestine. Add at least two ounces, and as much as eight to ten ounces of Noni to the colon-therapy machine. Perform the colonic irrigation as usual. Noni fruit juice added to a colonic irrigation can help the intestines feel soothed and peaceful, despite the relative stress of the colon therapy itself.

# -90-
# The Noni Gargle

## TRY THE NONI GARGLE
## THROAT CONDITIONS, INCLUDING:

- Dry throat.
- Sore throat.
- Strep throat.
- Tonsillitis.
- The onset of flu-like symptoms.

## HOW TO GARGLE WITH NONI:

1. Take a large sip of Noni fruit juice.

2. Gargle as usual. Allow the juice to gradually drip down your throat.

3. Continue gargling until you have swallowed all the Noni.

## MORE ABOUT THE NONI GARGLE:

Gargle as often as necessary throughout the day.

Try gargling with warm Noni Tea (page 185), which can also be soothing. However, most people prefer the feeling of cold Noni on their throats. The cold temperature adds an analgesic effect.

To do the Noni Gargle you could use some, or all, of the Noni that you would normally drink that day. However, if your throat is sore, you may need more Noni than usual. See the Procedure for Acute Conditions on page 75.

# -91-

# The Noni Gum Application

This procedure involves rubbing your gums with a cotton swab soaked in Noni.

## TRY THE NONI GUM APPLICATION
## FOR CONDITIONS SUCH AS:

- Gingivitis.
- Infected gums.
- Painful gums.
- Swollen gums.

## HOW TO DO THE NONI GUM APPLICATION:

1. Pour about one teaspoonful of Noni into a medicine cup or small bowl. Bring it with you into the bathroom.

2. Floss and brush your teeth as usual.

3. Dip one end of a cotton swab into the Noni juice. Rub this end of the swab against the affected gums.

4. Frequently dip the cotton swab back into the Noni to apply more juice to the gums. Continue until you have used up all of the Noni.

5. Follow with the Noni Mouthwash (page 363).

# MORE ABOUT THE
# NONI GUM APPLICATION:

Do this procedure at least once a day, or as often as necessary, until the condition improves.

The Noni Gum Application differs from the Noni Tooth and Gum Compress (page 383) because it requires you to rub the affected area rather than simply placing a compress pad there. Rubbing the area with the cotton swab increases circulation, which aids in the healing process and encourages the absorption of Noni's beneficial compounds.

As with all other Noni topical and internal applications, do this procedure at least three times before judging how well it is working for you.

# -92-

## The Noni Mouthwash

A refreshing and therapeutic alternative to the mint variety.

### USE NONI MOUTHWASH FOR:

- Bad breath.
- Cancer of the mouth.
- Gingivitis.
- Gum and mouth infections.
- Mercury poisoning that affects the gums, tongue or cheeks.
- Sores on the tongue, gums or inside the cheeks.
- Toothache.

### HOW TO USE NONI MOUTHWASH:

1. Take a relatively large sip of Noni fruit juice (about one to one-and-a-half teaspoonfuls). The juice will cause you to salivate.

2. Swish the Noni-saliva mixture around your teeth and gums and every corner of your mouth. If too much saliva is produced spit out some of the liquid. Continue to swish. Be careful not to swish too vigorously as the muscles in your mouth and tongue may feel sore afterward.

3. After about a minute, the flavor of the Noni will change.

This is an indication that your mouth has absorbed most of the Noni's beneficial compounds and may also have released toxins into the Noni. It is also a signal to spit out the Noni-saliva mixture.

## MORE ABOUT NONI MOUTHWASH:

Use the Noni Mouthwash two or three times daily, or as needed.

The swishing movement increases circulation and allows Noni to reach the entire mouth. It also incorporates air into the Noni-saliva mixture. The oxygen in this air is one of the reasons the Noni Mouthwash can make your mouth feel so good. The Noni helps carry the oxygen to the cells. This in turn activates the cells so they can receive even more of Noni's beneficial compounds.

You may gargle with the Noni Mouthwash, but gargle first, and then swish the Noni as described above.

A Noni Mouthwash can leave your teeth and gums feeling fresh and clean. It is a wonderful addition to your daily dental care routine.

If you are using the Noni Mouthwash for pain, you may feel relief immediately or soon afterwards. A few applications may be necessary to alleviate infection or other acute problems.

Chronic bad breath may require a daily Noni Mouthwash for a while, in addition to drinking Noni every day. Try Enhancing the Effects of Noni with Water on page 141 or the Procedure for Chronic Conditions on page 79.

The Noni Mouthwash is a less intense detoxification than the Oral Detox (page 371). The Noni Mouthwash helps draw toxins from the surface of the mouth, whereas the Oral Detox tends to draw toxins from deeper inside the tissues. Because the Noni Mouthwash helps draw out toxins from the mouth, try to avoid swallowing it. However, while you are swishing, it is natural to have an urge to swallow. It is possible to allow your body to have this reflex without actually swallowing very much Noni. This is easier to do if you lean forward when the throat muscles contract during the swallow reflex. Don't worry if a little juice drips down your throat.

If you are using the Mouthwash for mercury poisoning, take smaller sips and take extra care not to swallow any Noni. In addition, the flavor of the Noni may change sooner for you than for most other people, so you may swish for much less than a minute. You should also rinse your mouth with purified water after you spit out the liquid.

# -93-
## Noni Nose Drops

Noni Nose Drops can soothe the sinuses, reduce inflammation and ease congestion.

### USE NONI NOSE DROPS
### FOR CONDITIONS SUCH AS:

- Allergies that affect the sinuses.
- Colds and flu.
- Nasal infections.
- Nasal irritations.
- Sinusitis.
- Stuffy nose.

## HOW TO MAKE NONI NOSE DROPS:

1. Don't shake the Noni bottle before pouring the juice to make Noni Nose Drops. The watery portion of the juice, found at the top of an undisturbed bottle of Noni, is better for making Nose Drops (although it is not pulp-free). Because the Noni pulp may be mildly irritating, we'll also add some water to the Noni Nose Drops recipe as follows.

2. Pour one tablespoonful of Noni fruit juice into a small glass.

3. Add one tablespoonful of purified water. Let the Noni-water mixture rest for about five minutes so the pulp can settle to the bottom of the glass.

4. Carefully pour the top, pulp-free portion of the liquid into a drinking glass, small jar or tincture bottle with an eyedropper. You have now made Noni Nose Drops.

5. Drink the pulpy portion of the Noni-water mixture. Or use it to make two Noni Mini-compresses and place them on your sinuses after you have applied the Noni Nose Drops.

## HOW TO APPLY NONI NOSE DROPS:

**METHOD #1**
This is the easier of the two methods described in this chapter, but it requires a clean eyedropper.
1. Fill a clean eyedropper with Noni Nose Drops.

2. Hold the eyedropper in a cup of hot tap water to warm the Nose Drops.

3. Squeeze out a drop or two of Nose Drops onto the back of your hand. This serves two purposes: 1) it lets you test the temperature of the liquid, and 2) it removes any tap water that might have seeped into the eyedropper while warming it.

4. Lie down and tilt your head back. Insert a few drops of Noni Nose Drops into each nostril. Rest a few minutes while the Nose Drops seep into your sinuses. Have a paper napkin or paper towel handy for any Nose Drops that drip out when you get up.

**METHOD #2**

Use this method if you don't have an eyedropper. This method is not suggested for children because of the small size of their nostrils.

If you would like to warm the Nose Drops, use Method 1, 2, 3 or 4 described in the chapter titled, "Ways to Warm Noni" on page 405.

1.  Shape a piece of cotton ball into a cylinder about one inch long. It should be somewhat less wide than the diameter of your nostril's opening. Taper both ends of the cotton. Prepare a second piece of cotton the same way for your other nostril.

2.  Saturate one end of a cotton cylinder in the Noni Nose Drops solution.

3.  Lie down and tilt your head back. Have a paper towel or tissue handy to catch any Noni Nose Drops that may drip on your face.

4.  Insert the wet end of the cotton inside your nostril. At least half of the cotton should remain outside your nose.

5.  When you insert the cotton, some of the Noni Nose Drops will drip into your nose. To release more liquid from the cotton, gently press the side of your nose against the cotton that is inside it. You will feel the liquid drip into your sinuses.

6.  If you are performing the procedure on yourself, rest a few minutes before proceeding to the next step. If you get up too soon, the Nose Drops will drip out.

7. Repeat this procedure for the other nostril, using the second piece of cotton.

8. Again, rest a few minutes for the Nose Drops to seep into your sinuses.

## MORE ABOUT NONI NOSE DROPS:

Noni Nose Drops can be given as often as every few minutes to help clear and soothe the sinuses. Or, apply them a few times a day as needed.

Remember, Noni is a purple color and Noni Nose Drops may loosen and dissolve mucus. Don't be surprised when you blow your nose and see purple-stained mucus in the tissue paper.

Store Noni Nose Drops in a covered glass container in the refrigerator. The quantity of Noni Nose Drops solution suggested in the recipe on the previous page will be enough for several applications of Nose Drops. However, make a fresh batch each day you plan to use them. Use leftover Nose Drops to make Noni Mini-compresses to relieve your sinuses from the outside.

# -94-
# The Oral Detox

When Noni is held in prolonged contact with the roof of the mouth, Noni's restorative energies flood the head. This can be nourishing and can encourage detoxification.

## TRY THE ORAL DETOX
## FOR CONDITIONS IN THE:

- Brain.
- Ears.
- Eyes.
- Head.
- Mouth.
- Sinuses.
- Throat.

**As well as for:**

- Cancer.
- Chemical toxicity.
- Common cold.
- Cravings for nicotine, caffeine and other addictive substances.
- Depression.
- Earaches.
- Fever.
- Flu.
- Headaches.
- Heavy metal poisoning.
- Memory impairment.
- Mental illness.
- Sinusitis.

## HOW TO DO THE ORAL DETOX:

1. Take a small sip of Noni fruit juice.

2. Trap the Noni on top of your tongue and against the roof of your mouth. Do this by gently pressing the edges of your tongue against the inside of your upper teeth. This will also discourage saliva from mixing with the Noni, although some inevitably will.

3. Hold the sip in your mouth for about thirty to sixty seconds. Avoid swallowing the juice.

4. Spit out the Noni juice.

5. Rinse your mouth with purified water.

## MORE ABOUT THE ORAL DETOX:

Start by doing the Oral Detox once a day for about a week. Then try it twice a day if you are feeling well and think you can handle a stronger detoxification. If it is helpful, try the Oral Detox several times a day until symptoms abate.

If, during the Oral Detox, your mouth produces too much saliva to avoid swallowing, or if the Noni drips down your throat, spit some of it out. This will reduce the volume of liquid in your mouth. Next time take a smaller sip. Too much saliva mixed with the Noni will reduce the effectiveness of the Oral Detox procedure.

Even though you should hold the Noni against the roof of your mouth for 30 to 60 seconds, spit out the Noni sooner if you feel lightheaded or have any other uncomfortable reaction.

Every day, toxins and pollutants enter our body through our eyes, nose and mouth. They may be an underlying cause of common complaints such as headache, memory impairment, reduced mental clarity, "fuzzy" thinking, inability to stay focused, and attention deficit disorder. If you have these conditions, add the Oral Detox to your daily routine. For example, drink most of each daily serving that you usually take but save the last sip to use for the Oral Detox Procedure.

Do not underestimate the cleansing potential of the Oral Detox. If detoxification happens too quickly you may feel lightheaded, get a headache or experience other uncomfortable symptoms while doing the Oral Detox or soon afterwards. Drink plenty of purified water to help flush the toxins from your body. For other ideas about what to do during cleansing, refer to Appendix C, "Cleansing Reactions," on page 409. In addition, try the Noni Gentle Detoxification Program (page 181) and leave the Oral Detox for later.

On the other hand, the Oral Detox may ease head and mouth pain. It may also contribute to increased mental clarity and improved memory. Other beneficial "side-effects" can include relief from conditions such as gingivitis, toothache, mouth infections and oral sores.

# -95-
## The Noni Rectal Implant

Not a place you might expect to put a fruit juice! However, if you have problems here, you'll be glad you did.

### TRY THE NONI RECTAL IMPLANT FOR VARIOUS CONDITIONS OF THE RECTUM AND LOWER BOWEL:

- Cancer.
- Diverticulitis.
- Fissures.
- Hemorrhoids.
- Inflammation.
- Prostate cancer.

### HOW TO DO A NONI RECTAL IMPLANT:

1. Purchase a small disposable enema bottle from the drugstore. Open the bottle and pour the prepackaged liquid down the sink. Rinse out the bottle.

2. Pour one or two ounces of Noni fruit juice into the bottle and replace the bottle top. To warm the Noni, hold the bottle in a sink full of hot tap water.

3. Lubricate the bottle tip with an herbal ointment such as a comfrey or calendula salve. (Don't use petroleum jelly,

which will prevent Noni from reaching any area that the petroleum jelly covers, and don't use an ointment that contains menthol, for it will sting.)

4.  Find a comfortable position either lying on one side, lying on your back, bending over the sink or leaning over on your hands and knees. Insert the bottle tip into your rectum. Squeeze the bottle to release the Noni into your body.

5.  Hold the Noni in your body for as long as possible. Try to keep it in for at least five minutes. It is best to retain the Noni in your rectum until it is completely absorbed.

## MORE ABOUT THE
## NONI RECTAL IMPLANT:

If you have problems of the lower bowel and rectum, it is especially important to apply Noni there directly. When you drink Noni, its beneficial compounds spread throughout your body.  As the Noni passes through your digestive tract, the stomach and small intestines absorb the beneficial compounds. So not enough of them reach the lower bowel and rectum to be therapeutic—though the beneficial compounds will help your condition indirectly by uplifting your overall health.

Ideally, try to do the Noni Rectal Implant after you have taken an enema or have had a bowel movement. Then your rectum will be empty. If you take an enema beforehand, add a tablespoonful of Noni to the enema bag after filling it with warm water.  Doing so will soothe your intestines and introduce Noni beneficial compounds into the area.  It is important to expel as much of the enema into the toilet as possible before doing the Noni Rectal Implant. If too much water remains in your body, you may have a greater-than-usual urge to expel the Implant.

If you have an urge to expel the Noni Implant, try to keep it in for at least a few minutes, and then follow the urge. This urge may be your body's way of flushing toxins that the Noni has helped release. If your body has an immediate strong urge to expel the Implant, use less Noni next time.

If the rectum is highly irritated, the Noni might burn slightly at first. Soothing relief should soon follow.

Perform the Noni Rectal Implant daily. If your condition is relatively serious, gradually increase the amount of Noni in the Implant. You can use three to four ounces per application. (Disposable enema bottles usually hold up to four ounces of liquid.) When symptoms subside, gradually reduce the number of times you do the implant each week.

This procedure is suggested for prostate cancer because of the proximity of the prostate gland to the rectum. Cells in the rectum will spread Noni beneficial compounds to the nearby cells that need them most.

You can reuse the disposable enema bottle if you wash the bottle and the bottle tip with soap and water.

# -96-

## The Scent of Noni

### EMPLOY THE SCENT OF NONI TO:

- Focus the effects of Noni on conditions located inside the sinuses, brain and other organs in the head.
- Enhance the effects of Noni fruit juice, especially for conditions that stubbornly resist healing, and that are not responding to Noni fruit juice (or other methods).
- Invite the essence of Noni into your body in order to provide a pathway for Noni's beneficial compounds to reach more deeply into more cells.
- To uplift the health of the entire body.
- To clear the head for sharper thinking and memory.
- As an evaluation technique to find out how well your body may benefit from Noni.

### HOW TO EMPLOY
### THE SCENT OF NONI:

1. Pour one-half to one ounce of Noni fruit juice into a medicine cup.

2. Bring the medicine cup to your nose and deeply inhale Noni's aroma.

3. Move the cup away from your face and exhale through your mouth.

4. Repeat Steps 2 and 3 at least ten times or until you can no longer smell the aroma of Noni. This will occur when you have breathed in all the Noni molecules that you can absorb through your breath at this time.

## HOW TO USE THE SCENT OF NONI TO ENHANCE THE EFFECTS OF YOUR REGULAR SERVINGS OF NONI:

1. Pour your serving of Noni fruit juice into a medicine cup.

2. Bring the medicine cup to your nose and deeply inhale Noni's aroma.

3. Move the cup away from your face and exhale through your mouth.

4. Take a sip.

5. Repeat Steps 2, 3 and 4 until your serving is finished.

## MORE ABOUT THE SCENT OF NONI:

Raw Noni fruit has an unforgettable smell—in a word, it is nauseating. Fortunately, food scientists have been able to isolate the offending compounds, which have no therapeutic value, and remove them from Noni fruit juice. The juice still has an aroma, which is unique but not unpleasant.

The aroma of a substance consists of molecules of that substance radiating into the air. When you smell the scent of Noni, you are actually breathing in molecules of Noni. In other words, you are drinking in Noni's essence through your nostrils.

Enjoying the scent of Noni before you drink the juice has certain advantages. First, it prepares the body to accept Noni's beneficial compounds. Being given fair warning that a drink of Noni is coming, the body can better decide where to direct Noni's beneficial compounds. This is true whether you are taking Noni for the first time or have been drinking Noni for years.

The scent of Noni also introduces Noni to the brain. Making this introduction can be especially helpful when the body is hypersensitive to supplements, or tends to have strong cleansing reactions. After examining Noni's scent, the brain can evaluate whether Noni will be too strong or introduce changes too quickly. If the brain does come to this conclusion, then it will signal the body to repel Noni's scent, and this will discourage the individual from drinking the juice. In this case, if you still want to use Noni, it is better to apply it topically, or follow the Procedure to Gradually Introduce Noni to Your Diet (page 43), or the procedure for Enhancing Noni's Effects with Water (page 141), or Hydrating with Noni (page 145). Often the brain will signal the body to reject Noni if the body is dehydrated. So drinking extra water in this case would be suggested.

If you are a health professional dealing with people who are very sensitive, you can easily discover if Noni will help them— and even to what degree. Simply ask them to sample the scent of Noni as described in the steps above. If the scent pleases them, it is very likely Noni can help them a great deal. If they find the scent "okay," or "not offensive," then they can benefit from Noni, but maybe not dramatically so. An aversion to the scent of Noni can be a sign of toxicity or dehydration.

# -97-

# The Noni Tooth and Gum Compress

The mouth and gums seem to be more sensitive to Noni's analgesic properties than most other areas of the body.

## USE THE NONI TOOTH AND GUM COMPRESS FOR:

- Abscesses.
- Gum infection.
- Helping an area to heal after dental work.
- Helping to numb an area before dental work.
- Tooth infection and toothache.

## HOW TO MAKE AND APPLY THE NONI TOOTH AND GUM COMPRESS:

1. Make a Tooth and Gum Compress pad using either a cotton ball or gauze. If you use cotton, press it into a cylinder about two inches long and about one-half inch wide. If you use gauze, roll it into a cylinder of about the same size.

2. Turn a bottle of Noni upside down then right side up a few times to mix the pulp with the juice. Pour a teaspoonful of Noni fruit juice into a small bowl.

3. Press the compress pad into the Noni. Wipe up any pulp that remains in the bowl with the pulpy side of the compress pad.

4. Insert the wet compress pad into your mouth and onto the affected gums, with the pulpy side of the pad against the gums. It is okay to swallow any Noni fruit juice that leaks out.

5. Leave the compress pad in place for ten to fifteen minutes. By then much of the Noni fruit juice in the pad will have been swallowed and replaced by saliva. Even so, the pulp that clings to the compress pad would still be working.

6. Remove the compress pad and discard it.

7. Repeat the Noni Tooth and Gum Compress as often as needed.

## MORE ABOUT THE NONI TOOTH AND GUM COMPRESS:

Even if the pain is in a small area, make the compress pad about two inches long and apply it to the entire portion of the jaw where the pain is located. By using a relatively large compress pad, more of Noni's beneficial compounds will be absorbed into the area. You will then get the most benefit possible from Noni's analgesic properties.

Apply the Noni Tooth and Gum Compress both before and after any dental work you may receive. Doing the Compress beforehand can reduce any traumatic effects you may experience;

doing it afterwards can promote healing. Also, use the Noni Trauma Serving (page 95). It can help you relax and better handle the stress of visiting the dentist.

The Noni Tooth and Gum Compress can be used for tooth and gum conditions of all kinds. (For gum conditions, see also the Noni Gum Application on page 361.) However, if you have pain from a particular tooth, such as from an unfilled tooth cavity, infection or abscess, you may benefit from the following procedure:

1. Clean out the cavity with a toothbrush.

2. Apply the Noni Tooth and Gum Compress as outlined in Steps 1 through 4 above.

3. Dry the tooth with a clean cloth or piece of gauze.

4. Tear off a piece of a cotton ball large enough to cover the affected tooth. Soak the cotton in Noni fruit juice.

5. Press the Noni-soaked piece of cotton onto the tooth to fill the cavity with Noni. Bite and hold the cotton in place with the opposing teeth.

6. After ten to fifteen minutes, remove the cotton and the Noni Tooth and Gum Compress.

7. Repeat this procedure as often as needed.

# -98-
## Noni Toothpaste

Use Noni Toothpaste in addition to your regular daily dental hygiene program.

### USE NONI TOOTHPASTE:

- For daily oral hygiene.
- In addition to using your favorite toothpaste.

### HOW TO USE NONI TOOTHPASTE:

1. Pour about one teaspoonful of Noni fruit juice into a medicine cup and bring it with you to the bathroom.

2. Mentally divide your teeth into four quarters: upper-left, upper-right, lower-left and lower-right.

3. Dip your toothbrush into the Noni. Thoroughly brush the teeth and gums of one quarter of your mouth.

4. Spit out the juice. Rinse your toothbrush and tap out the excess water.

5. Repeat Steps 3 and 4 until you have brushed the teeth in all four quarters of your mouth.

## MORE ABOUT NONI TOOTHPASTE:

Noni Toothpaste leaves your teeth feeling clean. Since Noni does not contain the fluoride present in conventional toothpaste, it is important to brush with that as well, although at a different time.

In order to use Noni Toothpaste regularly, you will have to find a way to make the technique convenient. In temperate climates, you will be able to leave a few teaspoonfuls of Noni on the bathroom counter—enough for a few days—without the Noni spoiling. Otherwise, you could bring some Noni with you to the bathroom each day, although that may soon become bothersome. Or, leave an extra toothbrush near the kitchen sink and brush there daily with Noni.

# -99-
# The Noni Vaginal Implant

Noni can be implanted using a small disposable enema bottle, large plastic syringe tube—or even a turkey baster!

## USE THE NONI VAGINAL IMPLANT FOR VARIOUS CONDITIONS OF THE CERVIX, UTERUS, AND VAGINA, SUCH AS:

- Cervical cancer.
- Endometriosis.
- Uterine cancer.
- Uterine prolapse.
- Vaginitis.
- Yeast infections.

## HOW TO APPLY THE NONI VAGINAL IMPLANT:

1. Gather the things you will need to do the implant:
   - A pillow for your head.
   - A rolled up bath towel or another pillow to elevate your hips. (If you use a pillow, cover it with a towel.)
   - A feminine napkin.
   - A pantyliner for afterwards.
   - A small towel for cleaning.
   - Something to read to pass the time.

Use old towels, because Noni fruit juice will stain, and getting them wet is unavoidable.

2.  Add Noni fruit juice to a plastic syringe tube. This is the best kind of applicator because it allows you to control how much and how quickly you dispense the Noni. The standard amount for a Noni Vaginal Implant is one ounce.

3.  Lie on your back, with your hips on the pillow.

4.  Put the end of the applicator inside your body and slowly insert the Noni fruit juice. With your other hand, hold the feminine napkin under the syringe to catch any juice that spills. Try not to cough or sneeze, and try to relax your abdominal muscles. You'll soon discover how best to relax in order to retain as much of the Noni as possible.

5.  After you have inserted the Noni, remain lying in this position for about fifteen to twenty minutes.

6.  When you are ready to get up, hold the feminine napkin and the small towel between your legs to catch the juice. Most of it will spill out when you rise. Wear the panty-liner to collect any remaining Noni that may leak out later.

## MORE ABOUT THE
## NONI VAGINAL IMPLANT:

Do the Noni Vaginal Implant once a day. However, if the Implant results in foul odor, mucus discharge or tissue sloughing, this indicates the Noni is causing significant cleansing. In this case, do the Implant twice a day to support the vaginal detoxification.

You can find plastic syringe tubes at pet stores, especially those that specialize in large birds. (They are used to hand-feed large baby parrots.) Find a syringe that holds two ounces of liquid. The plunger in a one-ounce syringe tends to fall out when the syringe contains a full ounce of liquid; it can also be awkward to use.

An alternative to the plastic syringe tube is a disposable enema bottle that you can find at a drug store. Pour the contents of the bottle down the drain and rinse out the bottle. Pour an ounce of Noni into the bottle and replace the applicator top. Insert the applicator into your body, make sure the applicator is pointing down and squeeze the bottle gently. You may not need to warm the juice as you might for other topical and internal Noni applications because the vaginal tissue is less sensitive to temperature.

It may be more convenient to do the Vaginal Implant when you are in bed for the night. Then you can keep the Noni inside your body longer—at least until you get out of bed. Just keep your bed linens well protected and have old towels ready to catch the juice when you get up.

If you have a uterine prolapse, it will be difficult to implant much juice at first. Start with one-half ounce of Noni and work up to an ounce as the condition improves. Even if you use only one-half ounce of Noni, you may be able to insert only a small portion of this at a time. Hold as much of it inside you as you can; though it may leak right out, just insert a little more. Do this until you have used the entire half ounce of Noni.

The Noni Vaginal Implant can improve the health of the entire female reproductive system and may provide a pathway for toxins to leave the body. Therefore, although the Noni used in the Vaginal Implant won't come into direct contact with the ovaries, for example, the Vaginal Implant can still be helpful for conditions of the ovaries as well as for endometriosis. To help with pain, try daily applications of a Noni Poultice (page 229), the Noni Tummy Treatment #1 or #2 (page 337 and 341), Noni Paste (page 317), Noni Clay (page 251), or the Noni Abdominal Conditioner (page 235) over the painful areas.

# -100-
## The Noni Vaginal Tampon Implant

A quick and easy method to treat vaginal conditions.

### TRY THE NONI TAMPON IMPLANT FOR:

- Cervical conditions.
- Foul odor.
- Itchiness.
- Uterine conditions.
- Uterine prolapse.
- Vaginal conditions.
- Yeast infections.

### HOW TO APPLY
### THE NONI TAMPON IMPLANT:

1. Turn the Noni bottle upside and right side up a few times to mix the pulp with the watery portion of the Noni juice.

2. Pour one and one-half teaspoonfuls of Noni into a medicine cup. Take the medicine cup with you to the bathroom.

3. Unwrap a type of tampon called an O.B.® size regular. This type of tampon does not use an applicator.

4. Sit on the toilet seat.

5. Dip the end of the tampon into the Noni. It will quickly absorb the juice about halfway up the tampon. Use the wet end of the tampon to wipe up any pulp that remains in the medicine cup.

6. Insert the wet end of the tampon into your vagina.

## MORE ABOUT THE
## NONI TAMPON IMPLANT:

The advantage of the Noni Tampon Implant over the Noni Vaginal Implant is that you can keep Noni in contact with your body for a longer amount of time and you can easily reapply it several times a day. However, the Tampon Implant provides the area with a much smaller amount of Noni.

The Noni Tampon Implant may be preferred for those with uterine prolapse. When lying down, gently press the tampon into your body as far as it will go.

# -101-
## The Noni Vaginal Wipe

A fast and easy way to alleviate minor discomforts.

### WHEN TO USE THE
### NONI VAGINAL WIPE:

- After childbirth.
- For vaginal itching.
- For mild yeast infections.
- To freshen up after intercourse.
- To soothe chapped, irritated or dry labia.

### HOW TO APPLY THE
### NONI VAGINAL WIPE:

1. Dip a cotton ball in Noni fruit juice, so that only half of it gets wet.

2. Wipe the wet side of the cotton ball inside the vaginal opening. Then wipe between the labia. Squeeze the cotton ball as you apply it, or press it against your body to release the Noni onto your skin.

## MORE ABOUT THE
## NONI VAGINAL WIPE:

This procedure can be done after every urination, or as needed. Press the wet cotton against particularly sore or itchy areas to release the juice directly onto those areas.

Relief may come on contact with the Noni or several minutes later. Several applications may be needed. For more persistent conditions, apply a Noni Tampon Implant (page 393), or a Noni Compress (page 225) if the condition is focused on the labia.

After childbirth, your labia may be too tender to apply Noni with a cotton ball. Instead, add a tablespoonful or more of Noni to a sani-bottle that has been filled with warm distilled or purified water. After urinating, squirt the Noni-water mixture onto your labia. This can feel especially soothing.

# -APPENDIX A-

## WAYS TO ENHANCE THE EFFECTS OF NONI

Simply drinking a serving of Noni every day can improve your health and well-being, but there are times when you might want to enhance Noni's effects. Here is a list of Noni procedures that can help you get the best and the most out of every serving that you take.

### TRY ENHANCING THE EFFECTS OF NONI WHEN:

- You have health challenges that indicate taking more ounces of Noni than your body or your budget can handle.
- You are taking Noni for a particular condition and not getting the results you were hoping to achieve.
- Noni once helped a particular condition, but now your symptoms have returned even though you continue to take Noni.
- You have been taking Noni for a while and want to try some different ways to use Noni.

# HOW TO ENHANCE THE EFFECTS OF NONI:

The following techniques augment Noni's effects in various ways. Read the chapters listed and select a method that interests you and that might fit into your lifestyle. Then try it. In many cases, you can use more than one method at the same time.

**The Sipping Method to Find Your Ideal Amount** (page 55)
**The Noni Top Serving Procedure** (page 57):
These procedures can enhance Noni's effects by helping you find out exactly how much Noni your body really needs. When your body receives the right amount of Noni's beneficial compounds, it is in the best position to make healing changes.

**The Noni Anti-Stress Procedure** (page 119):
The techniques suggested in this procedure, including deep breathing and relaxation, allow the cells to better accept and utilize Noni's beneficial compounds.

**A Technique for Stubborn Conditions** (page 99):
This technique involves stimulating the cells by varying the amounts of Noni each day. This encourages the cells to recognize Noni's beneficial compounds and utilize them more effectively.

**Directing Noni with Breath and Focus** (page 123):
As the name of this procedure suggests, Noni's effects are enhanced with a special technique that directs Noni's beneficial compounds to those particular areas where you want them to work.

**The Busy Person's Way to Enhance their Daily Serving** (page 127):
This breathing technique helps your cells absorb Noni's beneficial compounds more effectively and efficiently by adding extra oxygen to the system.

**The Maintenance Economy Serving** (page 73)
**A Procedure for Serious Conditions #2** (page 87)
**Enhancing Noni's Effects with Water** (page 141):
These procedures enhance Noni's effects with water. Water transports Noni's beneficial compounds to the areas of the body that need them; it helps the cells take in the compounds they need and it helps the body flush toxins and wastes. Water enables Noni's beneficial compounds to spread throughout the body more quickly than drinking undiluted Noni. It also allows the cells to use Noni's beneficial compounds more effectively.

**Hydrating with Noni** (page 145):
This procedure helps your body use Noni's beneficial compounds more effectively by correcting dehydration. Dehydrated cells are inefficient at utilizing any health supplement, including Noni, and are unable to effectively absorb Noni's beneficial compounds.

**The Noni Chinese Body Clock Procedure** (page 109):
This procedure enhances Noni's effects by giving Noni to the body when certain organs are energetically most receptive to health and healing.

**Getting Comfortable with Noni** (page 69):
The ideas in this chapter show you how and when you can vary the ways you take Noni so that your body does not take the presence of Noni's beneficial compounds for granted. If this occurs, the cells will not use these compounds as efficiently as they could.

**Interrupting Your Noni Regimen** (page 105):
This procedure also asks your body not to take the presence of Noni's beneficial compounds for granted and teaches the body to not become dependent on Noni When you resume drinking Noni, the body usually responds by accepting Noni's beneficial compounds more efficiently and using them more effectively.

**Taking Noni with Herbs and Supplements** (page 137):
In general, healthful substances like vitamins, minerals, antioxidants, herbs and, of course, Noni, work synergistically to help the body become healthier. Taking these supplements at the same time can help them work better because the body receives all that it needs at once.

**Locating Noni's Target** (page 129):
This technique enhances Noni's effects through awareness. The rule is this: when you are aware of something and how it is working, it will work better.

**A Noni Detoxification Program** (page 177):
This procedure enhances Noni's ability to rid the body of toxins and wastes. It also strengthens the body and supports its immune system so that it can handle the cleansing more easily.

**Noni Tea** (page 185):
Noni's beneficial compounds support the immune system's natural ability to fight disease and infection. Noni Tea enhances this effect by highlighting one of the many restorative energies in Noni, which works to protect the body and strengthen its defense mechanisms.

**A Technique for Sharing Noni with Others** (page 217):
Drinking Noni with those who are enthusiastic about it can enhance the effects of Noni because of the positive atmosphere the group can generate. This will be true for those taking Noni for the first time, as well as those who have taken Noni for a long time. This is another good reason for family members to take their Noni at the same time. The love between family members lends a healing effect to anything they do together.

**The Auto-dilution** (page 133):
This procedure enhances the effects of Noni with your body's own life force. The Auto-dilution engages the body's awareness, wisdom and energetic pathways to take Noni's beneficial compounds and Noni's restorative energies to the precise locations in the body where they are needed most.

**The Scent of Noni** (page 379):
Inhaling the aroma of Noni prepares your brain and your body to receive and utilize the Noni beneficial compounds that you take into your body when you subsequently drink your Noni.

**SECTION 2 ON TOPICAL APPLICATIONS OF NONI:**
Use the topical and internal Noni applications that are appropriate for your condition. Doing so will support your condition by providing Noni's beneficial compounds exactly where they are needed. In particular:

**Noni Paste** (page 317):
You can enhance the topical effects of Noni by this cost effective way to concentrate Noni's beneficial compounds.

**Noni Clay** (page 251):
Clay enhances Noni's ability to detoxify the body.

**Noni for the Immune System** (page 305)
**The Noni Sitz Bath** (page 333):
When the entire body (or a large percentage of it), is covered with a health-promoting substance, its healing potential is stimulated and its energies are raised to a higher degree of vitality. This is why herbal baths can be so effective even when a relatively small amount of the herb or supplement is added to the bath.

**The Noni Abdominal Conditioner** (page 235)
**The Noni Tummy Treatment #1** (page 337)
**The Noni Tummy Treatment #2** (page 341):
Noni has an inherent ability to boost the immune system. Applying Noni to the abdomen is a way to stimulate the immune system using a topical method.

**Try Noni Liquid Concentrate:**
Enhance your experience of Noni with Noni liquid concentrate, which is available from most Noni distributors. Noni liquid concentrate supplies an abundance of Noni beneficial compounds; drop for drop, it contains much more than Noni fruit juice can supply on its own.

- Add a few drops of Noni liquid concentrate to your daily servings of Noni fruit juice.
- Rub a few drops of Noni liquid concentrate on areas associated with your health condition as well as areas of pain.
- Apply a few drops of Noni liquid concentrate to Noni fruit juice before you use the juice to make a topical application.
- Massage a few drops of Noni liquid concentrate on a target area before applying a topical application over it.
- Apply a few drops of Noni liquid concentrate to internal applications (except those used in the eyes and nose).

**Try Noni Seed Oil:**
Enhance your Noni juice experience with Noni seed oil, which is available from most Noni distributors. The rare Noni seed oil has a remarkable ability to penetrate the skin; carrying Noni's beneficial compounds with it. Noni seed oil should only be used topically.

- Rub a few drops of Noni seed oil on areas associated with your health condition as well as areas of pain.
- Massage a few drops of Noni seed oil on a target area before applying a topical application over it.
- Add a few drops of Noni seed oil to topical Noni formulas that include oil or lotion.
- Noni seed oil is convenient to carry with you and apply topically whenever you need the support of Noni beneficial compounds.

## MORE ABOUT ENHANCING
## THE EFFECTS OF NONI:

This chapter freely mentions, "enhancing the effects of Noni." To clarify, these techniques improve the body's ability to accept and respond to Noni's beneficial compounds. The body can become complacent and accustomed to anything that it receives regularly, including a health supplement like Noni. Varying the ways you use Noni and trying the techniques suggested in this chapter can help your body be as open and responsive as possible to Noni's healing potential.

# -APPENDIX B-

## WAYS TO WARM NONI FOR MORE COMFORTABLE TOPICAL AND INTERNAL APPLICATIONS

Noni fruit juice must be kept in the refrigerator to remain fresh. However, applying cold Noni to the body can sometimes be uncomfortable. Here are several ways to warm Noni for a more relaxing and inviting Noni experience.

### WARM NONI TOPICAL APPLICATIONS FOR:

- Infants and young children.
- Those who are very sick, weak and frail.
- The elderly.
- Those who are sensitive to cold.
- Conditions that would benefit from heat and warmth.
- Conditions that would be aggravated by cold temperature.

# WAYS TO WARM NONI:

## METHOD #1
Simply prepare the Noni application and keep it at room temperature until the refrigerated chill is gone. This method works particularly well in the summer.

## METHOD #2
1. Pour the Noni you want to use into a glass bowl.

2. Add a few inches of very hot tap water to the sink or to a large bowl.

3. Place the bowl with the Noni in the hot water. Be sure none of the water gets into the bowl.

4. When the heat of the hot water transfers through the glass bowl, it will also warm the Noni.

## METHOD #3
1. Pour boiling water into a glass bowl.

2. After about fifteen to thirty seconds, the heat from the water will transfer to the glass bowl. Pour out the water.

3. Quickly dry the bowl, which should still be hot, and pour in the amount of Noni you want to use. The heated bowl will warm the Noni.

## METHOD #4
1. Fill a glass bowl with hot tap water or heated water.

2. Pour the amount of Noni you want to use into a small plastic sandwich bag.

3.  Twist the open end of the bag so the Noni does not spill out.

4.  Hold the bag upright and submerge the end of the bag that contains the Noni under the hot water. Jiggle the bag so the heat can disperse through the Noni.

5.  Pour the Noni into a bowl and add the compress pad (or poultice pad, cotton ball or gauze).

**METHOD #5**

1.  Fill a glass bowl with hot water.

2.  Prepare the Noni compress pad (or poultice pad, cotton ball or gauze) per the instructions in the technique you want to try.

3.  Carefully put the Noni-soaked compress pad into a small plastic sandwich bag.

4.  Hold the bag upright and submerge the end of the bag that contains the Noni-soaked compress pad under the hot water.

See also "Ways to Heat Noni Poultices" (pages 233). Method #1 can be used for any application that involves mixing Noni with water. Method #2 can be used when you want a topical application that is as warm as you can get it without compromising Noni's beneficial compounds.

# MORE ABOUT WARMING
# NONI TOPICAL APPLICATIONS:

Warming is optional unless you want to employ heat to make the application more comfortable and/or to help the body absorb Noni's beneficial compounds.

Always test the temperature of heated Noni applications before applying them, especially to children.

Warmed Noni topical applications will cool after a while. To retain the warmth and collect body heat, cover the Noni application with a sheet of plastic wrap and then a folded towel.

Do not warm Noni in a microwave oven. This can destroy its beneficial compounds and will disrupt its restorative energies.

# -APPENDIX C-

# CLEANSING REACTIONS

Toxins are a part of life. They exist in our air, water and food and are also produced by the body as a result of normal functioning. The body naturally cleanses itself of toxins and metabolic wastes in many ways. However, a backlog often occurs. Toxins are stored and eventually they may contribute to disease. A healthy lifestyle supports the release of stored toxins. Sometimes, a healthful practice or supplement (like Noni) causes your body to release more toxins than your organs can handle at once. The symptoms that result are called a "cleansing reaction," "healing crisis" or "detoxification crisis."

Not everyone experiences cleansing reactions, no matter how much Noni they start out with. Moreover, sometimes when our body releases toxins we enjoy renewed health right away. This often results in what I call "positive cleansing reactions" (page 415).

This Appendix will help you identify cleansing reactions and give you some ideas about how to handle them.

# COMMON CLEANSING REACTIONS INCLUDE:

- Bad breath or body odor.
- Boils and pimples.
- Cough.
- Diarrhea or loose stools.
- Emotional releases.
- Foul-smelling urine.
- Headaches.
- Heavier-than-usual bleeding at menstruation.
- Intestinal gas or bloating.
- Joint pain (sudden onset, not due to injury).
- Mucus discharge.
- Skin rashes.
- Swollen glands.
- Unusual fatigue.

# HOW DO I KNOW IF I'M HAVING A CLEANSING REACTION?

Sometimes it can be difficult to know the difference between a cleansing reaction, an allergic reaction, hypersensitivity to Noni's beneficial compounds, or the symptoms of dehydration. The symptoms listed above may also indicate disease or illness, especially if they are longstanding. This chapter focuses on symptoms which occur suddenly, and which can be linked to taking Noni fruit juice.

**If you get a reaction after taking your first few servings of Noni:**
- You may have an allergy to Noni.

You should suspect an allergy to Noni if your symptoms begin after taking Noni the first time only, and if they include your body's typical responses to things you are allergic to. To find out if your reaction is an allergy, stop taking Noni, use the remedies that usually control your allergies, and wait until your symptoms subside. Then apply a Noni Mini-Compress (page 313) to your arm. If this gives you a rash or you get another sign of allergy, you probably are allergic to Noni. It may be best not to take Noni at this time.

• You might be hypersensitive to Noni's beneficial compounds. (In other words, taking too much stresses your body; a teaspoonful will do for you what one ounce might do for most other people.)

Suspect that this is the case if your symptoms do not include your body's typical responses to things you are allergic to. Your intuition might also let you know that you've taken too much Noni. Another way to find out if you are hypersensitive to Noni is to stop taking Noni and wait for your symptoms to subside. Then apply a Mini-compress to rule out allergy. If you do not get a rash or other allergic reaction, try other Noni topical applications. Give your body time to become accustomed to Noni. Try Gradually Introducing Noni to Your Diet (page 43).

• You are dehydrated.

This could be the case if you have been drinking fewer than two or three glasses of water a day. As a result, toxins have been building up in your body and Noni has suddenly invited them out. Most people need at least eight glasses of water a day to flush out metabolic wastes and toxins the body collects from food and the environment. If you are dehydrated and get symptoms that you suspect might be a cleansing reaction, simply drink more water. Your symptoms should go away rather quickly. If they do, continue to drink extra water. Try the procedures for Enhancing Noni's Effect with Water (page 141) and Hydrating with Noni (page 145).

In addition, sometimes dehydrated cells take in more Noni beneficial compounds than they should because the thirsty cells drink in the liquid that Noni fruit juice provides. In doing so, they also take in Noni beneficial compounds. If they take in more compounds than they can process because they lack enough water, bio-chemical imbalances can occur. The symptoms that result can seem like cleansing or allergic reactions, but are really evidence of this biochemical imbalance.

- You may indeed be having a cleansing reaction.

You should suspect that you're having a cleansing reaction if you have been taking Noni for a while without symptoms. Typical cleansing reactions often include foul odors, and they may or may not resemble your body's typical allergic responses. Cleansing reactions have no other explainable cause other than the healthful practice or supplement you have added to your lifestyle or whose amount or frequency you have recently increased. In hindsight, you can confirm a true cleansing reaction if, after the symptoms go away, you feel better than you did beforehand. After a cleansing reaction is over, you might also enjoy some degree of positive cleansing symptoms (page 415).

**If you have been taking Noni for a while, and then get cleansing symptoms:**
- You are probably not allergic to Noni or hypersensitive to its beneficial compounds, since you have been drinking Noni for a while without having had a reaction.

- You may be getting the flu or have the first symptoms of illness. See your doctor, especially if the symptoms do not go away after taking extra water to eliminate the possibility of dehydration.
- You may indeed be having a cleansing reaction.

**It can be hard to know if your symptoms are a result of a cleansing reaction or the flu because:**
- Both cleansing reactions and the flu tend to last the same amount of time.
- Both can be acute and short-lived; however, both can also drag out for some time.
- Natural methods for enhancing the immune system will help in either case.
- Antibiotics, cough suppressants and other pharmaceutical medicines often suppress a cleansing reaction. But they may be necessary to reduce symptoms and stabilize the body so it can gain strength for a more gradual detoxification later.

**You probably have a cold or flu if:**
You have been taking a Maintenance Serving of one ounce daily. Generally, one ounce a day of Noni is enough to supply the body's daily need for Noni's beneficial compounds. It is unlikely that this much Noni would initiate a cleansing reaction in most people.

**You are probably having a cleansing reaction if you are doing or have recently done the following:**
- The Top Serving Procedure.
- A Noni Fast.
- The Technique for Stubborn Conditions.
- A Noni Detoxification Program.
- A Noni Protocol to Quit Smoking and for Addiction Relief.

- Changed the amount of your daily serving.

> Please see a Health Professional if your symptoms become more than you can comfortably address with home remedies.

## WHAT TO DO IF YOU THINK YOU ARE HAVING A CLEANSING REACTION:

Cleansing reactions are ultimately helpful to the body, though they can be uncomfortable. Do what you can to clear your body of the toxins it is trying to release. For example:

- Give yourself extra time to rest and sleep.
- Make sure you drink at least eight glasses of purified water a day. Water is essential to flush toxins from the system.
- Substitute a serving of Noni Tea (page 185) for each serving of Noni that you usually take.
- Drink an extra serving or two of Noni in the form of Noni Tea.
- Try taking the same number of daily servings as usual, but take only half the amount of Noni in each serving. Drinking less Noni during a cleansing reaction can slow the release of toxins.
- Take each of your servings in the form of an Auto-dilution (page 133).
- Use the Noni Tummy Treatment either in place of your regular Noni servings or in addition to them.
- Try the Noni Abdominal Conditioner (page 235) and Noni for the Immune System (page 305).
- Try drinking a half a glass of water both before and after your serving of Noni. This will encourage

Noni's beneficial compounds to enter your body more gradually—with less immediate impact. Those who feel that their body is particularly toxic can try this technique with every serving of Noni that they take, in order to encourage a more gradual detoxification.

- Try the Noni Fast Method #2 (page 175), Enhancing Noni with Water (page 141), or Hydrating with Noni (page 145).
- Combine Noni fruit juice with other modalities. Noni is compatible with all natural healing methods, including herbs, homeopathic remedies, chiropractic, Chinese Medicine, Ayurvedic Medicine, Bach flower essences, vitamins and minerals, chelation therapy, acupuncture, massage and others.

In general, any reaction to Noni is better than no reaction at all. The reaction proves that your body recognizes Noni and that Noni can indeed help you. After the cleansing reaction is over, reevaluate the procedure for drinking Noni that you were using. You may want to stick with it, now that you have reached a higher level of health. Or you may want to make some changes in your drinking procedure and serving size.

## POSITIVE CLEANSING REACTIONS:

Although cleansing reactions have a reputation for being unpleasant, they can also produce positive symptoms such as those below. Unfortunately, positive cleansing reactions don't last as long as we would like them to. Positive reactions almost always occur within the first few days or weeks after you add a health-supporting supplement like Noni to your diet, or after Interrupting Your Noni Regimen (page 105), or even after you've had a true cleansing reaction.

**Positive Reactions Can Include:**
- Significantly improved memory.
- Remarkably clearer thinking.
- A surge of creativity and new ideas.
- A greater sense of well-being.
- More energy and clarity than usual.
- Insights into the purpose and meaning of life.
- Dreams that are more meaningful and easier to remember.
- A sudden ability to see the overview of life itself, or of various situations that we may be involved with.
- Unusual hypersensitivity to one's own thoughts, needs and feelings, as well as to those of others.
- A great deal of excitement and enthusiasm for Noni.

Any degree of the above experiences may be considered a positive cleansing reaction if the experience is obviously connected to taking Noni.

Naturally, we welcome the positive cleansing reactions, but try not to be disappointed when they go away. Your body will soon adjust to a greater level of health, and the positive reactions will lessen as you settle into a new, healthier state of "normal." Continue to take Noni to maintain your journey to greater health.

## MORE ABOUT CLEANSING REACTIONS:

Old injuries, health challenges, and particularly intense emotions may also surface briefly, and are indicators of a kind of cleansing reaction. Old injuries and conditions tend to arise in reverse order, as progressively older conditions are re-experienced. They will soon pass if their healing process is given adequate support. Be sure to address them with the appropriate topical and internal Noni applications, in addition to your daily oral servings of Noni.

Loose stools tend to occur when you are taking more Noni than you need. This may occur, for example, if you are a nursing mother taking extra Noni for a sick baby. The Noni you drink will pass into your breastmilk. You will have to weigh the benefits of the Noni for your baby against the relative inconvenience of frequent visits to the bathroom. If your baby gets loose stools, however, then you know you are taking too much.

Ideally, Noni should allow you to detoxify gradually and feel good at the same time. Then, if you do have a cleansing reaction, adjusting the amount of Noni you take and how you take it can help you detoxify more comfortably.

# -APPENDIX D-

# WHAT IF NONI DOESN'T SEEM TO WORK FOR ME?

If Noni doesn't seem to be helping or isn't working as fast as you would like, ask yourself the following questions. The answers may help you understand what may be happening, and give you some ideas about what to do.

## FOR WHAT CONDITION ARE YOU TAKING NONI?

It helps to decide why you are taking Noni. This makes it easier to correlate Noni's effects with changes in your health. Use the information and charts in the chapters: Noni Health Evaluation Sheets (page 17), Evaluating your Progress with Noni (page 25), How to Achieve your Health Goals with Noni (page 29) and Using Intention with Noni (page 115).

## HAVE YOU FILLED OUT THE HEALTH EVALUATION SHEET #2? (PAGES 22-23)

If you have not, maybe now is the time to do so. Compare your symptoms now with how you felt when you filled out Sheet #1. If you have not filled out either sheet, try to remember what your condition was like before you started to drink Noni. Write down what symptoms you had. How severe were they? Take an honest look at how you feel now. Is there any difference at all? Ask a friend or family member to recall your state of health and well-being before you began taking Noni, and to evaluate your health as it is now. This feedback will be invaluable. In fact, it can be more helpful than your own evaluation in deciding how well Noni is working for you.

## HOW LONG HAVE YOU HAD THIS CONDITION?

If your condition is chronic and long-standing, you may need more time on any health improvement program before you see results. In the process of healing, healthier cells replace sick or damaged cells. This always seems to take longer than one would like. You probably won't feel a difference in your health until enough of these cell replacements have occurred.

## HOW LONG HAVE YOU BEEN DRINKING NONI?

In some cases, it can take several months before you enjoy positive changes in your health. Give Noni a fair chance to work, and give yourself a fair opportunity to heal.

## HOW MUCH NONI FRUIT JUICE ARE YOU TAKING?

Some people's bodies need more Noni than others do, even for maintenance. In general, the more serious the condition the more Noni you may need.

## ARE YOU TAKING NONI FRUIT JUICE REGULARLY?

When addressing any health condition with Noni fruit juice, it is important to take your servings regularly. Make sure you have enough juice on hand so you won't run out.

## HAVE YOU NOTICED ANY UNEXPECTED CHANGES IN YOUR HEALTH?

Have you noticed any improvement in minor discomforts? It is easy to overlook these kinds of improvements, especially if you are taking Noni for a major health challenge. (For example, I had no idea my eyesight had improved until someone mentioned that theirs had. I may never have noticed otherwise!)

## HAVE YOU HAD ANY CLEANSING REACTIONS SINCE YOU STARTED TAKING NONI?

For a list of common cleansing reactions, see page 410. Cleansing reactions, though generally uncomfortable, should be considered beneficial because they signal that the body is experiencing a major cleansing. Detoxification is often a necessary first step before cell repair and health building can begin.

## DID NONI EVER WORK FOR YOU AT ALL?

There is a difference between the experience of not ever having noticed any effects from Noni at all, either positive or negative, and the experience of noticing a difference at first, and then nothing thereafter. If you have never, ever noticed anything from Noni, and you have been taking Noni for at least a few months, then perhaps your body simply doesn't need Noni's beneficial compounds. Or maybe your body doesn't know how to put these compounds to good use. If you noticed a difference at first, and then nothing since, you know that Noni can help you. It may now be working below the threshold of your ability to perceive its effects. Or, it may be helping you to maintain your present level of health, and preventing it from getting worse. Try the techniques in Appendix A, "Ways to Enhance the Effects of Noni," (page 397).

## WHAT ABOUT POSITIVE CHANGES IN YOUR PERSONALITY, EMOTIONS, MENTAL CLARITY, OR MEMORY?

Sometimes Noni seems to work on our non-physical aspects first. We may become more patient, calm, joyful, better able to handle stress and emotions, or perhaps less irritable, impatient or moody. Don't overlook these other possible benefits.

**ARE YOU TAKING OTHER HEALTH SUPPLEMENTS?**
Noni is not a cure-all. Although Noni provides important micronutrients, it does not supply all the nutrition that the body needs. It is possible that your condition would benefit from other supplements. Try a full-spectrum vitamin and mineral supplement that would help meet all your nutrient requirements.

**WHAT ACTIVITIES DO YOU NOW ENJOY SINCE YOU BEGAN TO TAKE NONI?**
Sometimes the best gauge of improved health is not how we feel, but how well we can enjoy life.

# -APPENDIX E-

## WHAT IF MY SYMPTOMS RETURN?

Some people find that after Noni alleviates certain symptoms, these symptoms eventually return. It is tempting to say that Noni has stopped working. But this is not necessarily the case. Here are a few possible explanations, plus some ideas for how you can use Noni if your symptoms do come back.

- Many people who start taking Noni say they feel better almost right away. They may be experiencing positive cleansing reactions (page 415), which may be making them feel so good, they don't notice their symptoms. Unfortunately, their symptoms will probably "return" when the positive cleansing reactions no longer mask them. Lasting positive changes in one's health won't occur until they are supported by actual changes in the cells. These changes usually take time.

- After taking Noni, many people find they can eat foods that once before caused certain symptoms such as indigestion, headaches, or joint pain. They find they can work harder, play harder, go to bed later and get up earlier, too. Instead of using Noni's beneficial compounds to help us grow healthier, we often use them to help us get away with doing things that are less healthy (albeit enjoyable). There is nothing wrong with this. But if we abuse the freedom, it won't last. When the body can no longer handle the added stress, we will again need more sleep and favorite foods will again cause discomfort. Symptoms may appear to return, when really they weren't given the opportunity to heal in the first place.

- The body will continue to age and manifest stress at its weakest points, no matter how wonderful the therapies that we give to it. If new stresses are introduced into our lives, these weakest points may again reveal themselves and conditions that were once alleviated may return.

- During the healing process, pain and other symptoms may go away. But this doesn't mean our ailment is cured. It can take a while for healthy cells to replace unhealthy cells. Meanwhile, we may become more active than before and cause additional stress on the healing tissue. Symptoms may return, simply to remind us to take better care of ourselves.

- Health improves in cycles: A period of health building follows every period of well-being. This health-building period may pass unnoticed or make us feel more tired than usual. Or it may include an intense cleansing, when the body releases toxins, wastes, fat, and various excesses that it may have been storing. As these toxins enter the bloodstream, they pass by our weak or problem areas. These toxins can irritate these areas, causing symptoms to temporarily resurface or worsen.

- Symptoms can be signals to take better care of ourselves. Recurring symptoms may be our body's best way to tell us we need something that we have not yet given to our body. Perhaps we need more rest, or a nutrient that is missing from our diet.
- Recurring symptoms may also alert us to look at our

condition from another angle. Perhaps there are mental or emotional causes that we have been overlooking. Sometimes physical improvement cannot continue until we take care of the mental and emotional aspects of ourselves.

- Dr. Ralph Heinicke offered yet another explanation for why symptoms may return in a letter he wrote to me in October, 1997. He writes, "I now believe that some people have a marginal supply of several crucial micronutrients. Initially proxeronine is the limiting factor. This explains the tremendous response [from taking Noni] which some people observe. However, after taking Noni for a while, other micronutrients become limiting factors for good health."

  Dr. Heinicke then offers two approaches, "1) to discover what the next specific health limiting factor is, or 2) to take a supplement which contains a wide variety of potentially limiting factors."

Returning symptoms often go away again after Interrupting Your Noni Regimen (page 105) for a few days. In fact, after resuming Noni, health sometimes takes a leap for the better. Here are some ideas that may explain why Interrupting Your Noni Regimen works:

- Symptoms may return if the body becomes accustomed to Noni's beneficial compounds. To obtain the same results as before, the body would need greater amounts of Noni. Taking larger servings may indeed help for a while. Interrupting Your Noni Regimen seems to readjust the body's relationship to Noni's beneficial compounds so the smaller amounts of Noni become helpful again.

- The cells in our bodies are innately intelligent, and like us, they have a memory and can take on both good and bad habits. As new cells replace old cells, the new cells may not remember how conditions once were without Noni. They may take the now-constant supply of Noni's beneficial compounds for granted and not use them as best as they can. Interrupting Your Noni Regimen encourages the cells to use these compounds more effectively and efficiently.

- Another possibility is that when certain unused Noni compounds are stored in the body for too long, they may start to cause stress. Perhaps they deteriorate into other compounds. If this is so, maybe Interrupting Your Noni Regimen clears out the old stores. Then Noni usually works just as well as, if not better than it did before.

If your symptoms return, but it is not appropriate to Interrupt Your Noni Regimen because you have immune deficiency conditions, diabetes, cancer or a life-threatening condition, here are some techniques you could try:

- Take sips of your servings on a regular time schedule. For example, take a sip every five, fifteen, or sixty minutes. Set a timer to ensure you keep to the rhythm.
- Try the Auto-dilution (page 133) and the Noni Tummy Treatments (pages 337 and 341).
- Also try other topical and internal Noni applications that are appropriate for your condition.
- Try Sipping (page 39) your servings of Noni if you usually drink them All at Once (page 41), or vice versa.
- Try the techniques in Appendix A, "Ways to Enhance the Effects of Noni" (page 397).
- Examine your diet and lifestyle. Are you taking part in

any activities that might be stressing your body? Find out what foods you may be allergic to, and eliminate them from your diet. Some health practitioners have ways to test for allergies, which can give you immediate feedback. Get more rest, try meditation or spiritual exercise, and take better care of yourself emotionally, mentally, physically and spiritually.

# -INDEX-

Noni Tooth and Gum Compress 6, 362, 383, 384, 385

Noni to Enhance Dreams and Sleep 261

Noni to help lose weight 64

Noni Vaginal Tampon Implant 393

Noni Vaginal Wipe 6, 395

Noni's effectiveness *k*

Noni's beneficial compounds 2, 8, 9, 44, 45, 60, 65, 77, 83, 88, 89, 90, 105, 106, 107, 108, 117, 123, 124, 125, 128, 135, 138, 139, 141, 142, 143, 145, 148, 149, 156, 157, 167, 170, 185, 186, 189, 192, 194, 208, 223, 227, 230, 231, 233, 237, 250, 266, 267, 274, 275, 278, 279, 283, 286, 310, 311, 316, 320, 324, 339, 340, 362, 364, 379, 381, 384, 398, 399, 400, 401, 402, 403, 407, 408, 410, 411, 413, 415, 421, 423, 425, 426

Noni's restorative energies 2, 135, 231, 263, 266, 371, 401

North American Indians 245

Nose Drops *i*, 186, 367, 368, 369, 370

nursing mother 83, 417

nutrient-depleted soils *d*

nutrients *e*, 3, 48, 63, 116, 125, 136, 167, 238, 242, 273

nutritional deficiency 13, 47

nutritional supplements i, 48, 131

## O

old injuries 229, 416, 417

opportunities 6

Oral Detox 6, 131, 135, 159, 168, 364, 371, 372, 373

oral hygiene 387

oral sores 373

organic material *k*

organ failure 83

otoscope 353

ovaries 235, 391

over-stressed nervous system 263

overall condition 213

overall health 3, 29, 80, 121, 269, 376

overeating 195

oxygen 12, 125, 128, 364, 398

oxygen molecules 128

## P

pain *i*, 20, 22, 39, 41, 42, 79, 95, 96, 107, 140, 145, 232, 237, 239, 241, 242, 247, 249, 250, 251, 254, 256, 258, 269, 271, 277, 278, 279, 282, 283, 284, 285, 293, 300, 303, 305, 309, 317, 320, 321, 341, 349, 353, 364, 373, 384, 385, 391, 402, 403, 410, 423, 424

painful areas 225, 229, 237, 241, 321, 391

painful gums 361

painful joints 323

painkilling elements *k*

pancreas 112, 124, 229, 235, 237

parasites 44, 45, 57, 171, 173, 181, 237, 238, 341, 355, 357

pathway for Noni's beneficial compounds 379

performance 1, 57, 59, 60, 170, 200, 213

personal choices *c*

personal hygiene 347

personal power c

pets 207, 211, 213, 349

pharmaceutical companies  c
pharmaceutical medicines  413
phase of positive change  41
phosphorus  274
physicians  c, d
physiological need  152, 167
phytonutrients  c
pimples  227, 245, 273, 313, 325,
    327, 335, 410
pinched nerves  247
pineal gland  12, 170, 263
pinkeye  265, 269
plastic syringe  j, 208, 209, 210,
    213, 389, 390, 391
plastic syringe tubes  208
plateau  13, 59, 99, 105
PMS  75, 79, 348
poison ivy  77, 323, 325, 327, 335
Polynesians  274
Polynesian islands  g
poor circulation  287, 291
poor eating habits  171
positive changes  42, 420, 423
positive cleansing reactions  409,
    415, 416, 423
posture  219, 250
potassium  148
poultice pads  227, 228
pre-cancerous cells  k
pregnancy  i, 145
pregnant mothers  105
premature labor contractions  i
prescription medications  31, 43, 46,
    140, 169, 170
prevent disease  207
prevent injuries  225
Procedure for Serious Conditions #1
    83, 84
Procedure for Serious Conditions #2
    87, 88

Procedure for Acute Conditions  75
Procedure for Chronic Conditions
    79
Procedure for Life-Threatening
    Conditions  91
Procedure for Serious Conditions  j,
    84, 87, 88, 89, 93, 99, 143,
    162, 163, 399
profound sadness  133
prostate cancer  375, 377
prostate conditions  139
prostate gland  139, 377
protein  k, 3, 172, 173, 176, 231
protein molecules  173, 231
Protocol to Quit Smoking and for
    Addiction Relief  151
proxeronine  k, 3, 425
psoriasis  325, 329, 335
psychological need  159
pulp  7, 193, 226, 230, 235, 242,
    249, 252, 265, 266, 270, 271,
    273, 278, 295, 297, 299, 300,
    305, 307, 310, 314, 318, 320,
    334, 336, 338, 352, 353, 367,
    368, 383, 384, 393, 394
puncture wounds  313
pure extract  g
purified water  47, 49, 93, 137, 142,
    166, 171, 172, 175, 185, 227,
    229, 230, 251, 261, 265, 269,
    277, 335, 347, 355, 365, 368,
    372, 373, 414
purpose  m, 13, 81, 271, 339, 416
pus  233

## Q

questionnaire  17
Quick Noni Paste  6, 314, 323, 324